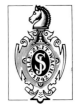

World Health Organization

The series *International Histological Classification of Tumours* consists of the following volumes. Each of these volumes – apart from volumes 1 and 2, which have already been revised – will appear in a revised edition within the next few years. Volumes of the current editions can be ordered through WHO, Distribution and Sales, Avenue Appia, CH-1211 Geneva 27.

1. Histological typing of lung tumours (1967, second edition 1981)
2. Histological typing of breast tumours (1968, second edition 1981)
3. Histological typing of soft tissue tumours (1969)
4. Histological typing of oral and oropharyngeal tumours (1971)
5. Histological typing of odontogenic tumours, jaw cysts, and allied lesions (1971)
6. Histological typing of bone tumours (1972)
7. Histological typing of salivary gland tumours (1972)
8. Cytology of the female genital tract (1973)
9. Histological typing of ovarian tumours (1973)
10. Histological typing of urinary bladder tumours (1973)
12. Histological typing of skin tumours (1974)
13. Histological typing of female genital tract tumours (1975)
14. Histological and cytological typing of neoplastic diseases of haematopoietic and lymphoid tissues (1976)
16. Histological typing of testis tumours (1977)
17. Cytology of non-gynaecological sites (1977)
20. Histological typing of tumours of the liver, biliary tract and pancreas (1978)
21. Histological typing of tumours of the central nervous system (1979)
22. Histological typing of prostate tumours (1980)
23. Histological typing of endocrine tumours (1980)
24. Histological typing of tumours of the eye and its adnexa (1980)
25. Histological typing of kidney tumours (1981)

A coded compendium of the International Histological Classification of Tumours (1978).

The following volumes have already appeared in a revised edition with Springer-Verlag:
Histological Typing of Thyroid Tumours, 2nd edn. Hedinger/Williams/Sobin (1988)
Histological Typing of Intestinal Tumours, 2nd edn. Jass/Sobin (1989)
Histological Typing of Oesophageal and Gastric Tumours, 2nd edn. Watanabe/Jass/Sobin (1990)
Histological Typing of Tumours of the Gallbladder and Extrahepatic Bile Ducts, 2nd edn. Albores-Saavedra/Henson/Sobin (1990)
Histological Typing of Tumours of the Upper Respiratory Tract and Ear, 2nd edn. Shanmugaratnam/Sobin (1991)

In this series, colour illustrations will be limited in number in order to maintain a reasonable sales price. The present volume is an exception owing to contributions obtained by the author.

A set of 200 colour slides (35 mm), corresponding to the photomicrographs in the book, is available from the American Registry of Pathology, 14th Street and Alaska Ave. NW, Washington, DC 20306, USA. For further information please see p. 201.

Histological Typing of Tumours of the Upper Respiratory Tract and Ear

K. Shanmugaratnam

In Collaboration with L. H. Sobin
and Pathologists in 8 Countries

Second Edition

With 200 Figures

Springer-Verlag
Berlin Heidelberg New York
London Paris Tokyo
Hong Kong Barcelona
Budapest

K. Shanmugaratnam
Head, WHO Collaborating Centre
for the Histological Classification
of Upper Respiratory Tract Tumours
Department of Pathology
National University of Singapore
Republic of Singapore

L. H. Sobin
Head, WHO Collaborating Centre
for the International Histological Classification
of Tumours
Armed Forces Institute of Pathology
Washington, DC, USA

First edition published by WHO in 1978 as No. 19 in the International Histological Classification of Tumours series

ISBN 3-540-53880-1 Springer-Verlag Berlin Heidelberg New York
ISBN 0-387-53880-1 Springer-Verlag New York Berlin Heidelberg

Library of Congress Cataloging-in-Publication Data
Shanmugaratnam, K. Histological typing of tumours of the upper respiratory tract and ear / K. Shanmugaratnam; in collaboration with L. H. Sobin and pathologists in 8 countries. – 2nd ed. p. cm. – (International histological classification of tumours) Rev. ed. of: Histological typing of upper respiratory tract tumours. 1978. Includes bibliographical references and index.
ISBN 3-540-53880-1 (alk. paper). –
ISBN 0-387-53880-1 (alk. paper)
1. Respiratory organs–Tumors–Histopathology. 2. Ear–Tumors–Histopathology. 3. Tumors–Classification. I. Shanmugaratnam, K. Histological typing of upper respiratory tract tumours. II. Sobin, L. H. III. Title. IV. Series: International histological classification of tumours (Unnumbered) [DNLM. 1. Ear Neoplasms– classification. 2. Ear Neoplasms-pathology. 3. Respiratory Tract Neoplasms-classification. 4. Respiratory Tract Neoplasms-pathology. WF 15 S528h] RC280.R38S52 1991 616.99'2207583-dc20 DNLM/DLC for Library of Congress 91-4840 CIP

© Springer-Verlag Berlin Heidelberg 1991
Printed in Germany

The use of general descriptive names, registered names, trademarks, etc. in this publication does not imply, even in the absence of a specific statement, that such names are exempt from the relevant protective laws and regulations and therefore free for general use.

Product liability: The publishers cannot guarantee the accuracy of any information about dosage and application contained in this book. In every individual case the user must check such information by consulting the relevant literature.

Reproduction of the figures: Gustav Dreher GmbH, Stuttgart
Typesetting and printing: Appl, Wemding; Binding: Schäffer, Grünstadt
21/3145-543210 – Printed on acid-free paper

Participants

Barnes, L., Dr.
Division of Head and Neck Pathology, Presbyterian University
Hospital, Pittsburg, USA

Cardesa, A., Dr.
Catedratico de Anatomia Patologica, Facultad de Medicina,
Barcelona, Spain

Ferlito, A., Dr.
Institute of Otorhinolaryngology, University of Padua, Padova, Italy

Friedmann, I., Dr.
Northwick Park Hospital & Clinical Research Centre, Middlesex,
UK

Heffner, D. K., Dr.
Department of Otolaryngic Pathology, Armed Forces Institute
of Pathology, Washington, DC, USA

Hellquist, H. B., Dr.
Head & Neck Unit, Orebro Medical Center Hospital, Orebro,
Sweden

Hyams, V. J., Dr.
Department of Otolaryngic Pathology, Armed Forces Institute
of Pathology, Washington, DC, USA

Krueger, G. R. F., Dr.
Pathologisches Institut, Universität zu Köln, Köln,
Federal Republic of Germany

Micheau, C., Dr.
Department d'Anatomie Pathologique, Institut Gustave-Roussy,
Villejuif, France

Nascimento, A., Dr.
Dept Patologia, Instituto Nacional de Cancer, Rio De Janeiro,
Brazil

Shanmugaratnam, K., Dr.
Department of Pathology, National University of Singapore,
Republic of Singapore (WHO Collaborating Centre for the
Histological Classification of Upper Respiratory Tract Tumours)

Sobin, L. H., Dr.
Armed Forces Institute of Pathology, Washington, DC, USA
(WHO Collaboration Centre for the International Histological
Classification of Tumours)

General Preface to the Series

Among the prerequisites for comparative studies of cancer are international agreement on histological criteria for the definition and classification of cancer types and a standardized nomenclature. An internationally agreed classification of tumours, acceptable alike to physicians, surgeons, radiologists, pathologists and statisticians, would enable cancer workers in all parts of the world to compare their findings and would facilitate collaboration among them.

In a report published in 1952,[1] a subcommittee of the World Health Organization (WHO) Expert Committee on Health Statistics discussed the general principles that should govern the statistical classification of tumours and agreed that, to ensure the necessary flexibility and ease of coding, three separate classifications were needed according to (1) anatomical site, (2) histological type, and (3) degree of malignancy. A classification according to anatomical site is available in the International Classification of Diseases.[2]

In 1956, the WHO Executive Board passed a resolution[3] requesting the Director-General to explore the possibility that WHO might organize centres in various parts of the world and arrange for the collection of human tissues and their histological classification. The main purpose of such centres would be to develop histological definitions of cancer types and to facilitate the wide adoption of a uniform nomenclature. The resolution was endorsed by the Tenth World Health Assembly in May 1957.[4]

---

[1] WHO (1952) WHO Technical Report Series. No. 53, 1952, p 45
[2] WHO (1977) Manual of the international statistical classification of diseases, injuries, and causes of death. 1975 version Geneva
[3] WHO (1956) WHO Official Records. No. 68, p 14 (resolution EB 17.R40)
[4] WHO (1957) WHO Official Records. No. 79, p 467 (resolution WHA 10.18)

Since 1958, WHO has established a number of centres concerned with this subject. The result of this endeavour has been the International Histological Classification of Tumours, a multivolumed series whose first edition was published between 1967 and 1981. The present revised second edition aims to update the classification, reflecting progress in diagnosis and the relevance of tumour types to clinical and epidemiological features.

Preface to Histological Typing of Upper Respiratory Tract Tumours, Second Edition

The first edition of *Histological Typing of Upper Respiratory Tract Tumours*[1] was the result of a collaborative effort organized by WHO and carried out by the International Reference/Collaborating Centre for the Histological Classification of Upper Respiratory Tract Tumours at the Department of Pathology of the National University of Singapore. The Centre was established in 1972, and the classification was published in 1978.

In order to keep the classification up to date, the Centre invited proposals for revision from the participating pathologists listed on pages V and VI. Their responses provided the basis for the preparation of a revised classification. Drafts of the definitions and explanatory notes prepared at the Centre were circulated among all participants, and their comments were taken into account in the preparation of this volume. There were a few tumour types on which the participants expressed divergent views on the classification, terminology or definition. In such cases this volume expresses the views of the majority of participants with due regard to consistency with other volumes in this series. It will, of course, be appreciated that the classification reflects the present state of knowledge, and modifications are almost certain to be needed as experience accumulates. It is therefore expected that some pathologists may wish to dissent from certain aspects of the classification or terminology adopted in this volume. It is nevertheless hoped that, in the interests of international cooperation and comparability of data, all pathologists will use the classification as put forward. Criticisms and suggestions for its improvement will be welcomed; these should be sent to the World Health Organization, Geneva, Switzerland.

---

[1] Shanmugaratnam K, Sobin LH (1978) Histological Typing of Upper Respiratory Tract Tumours. Geneva, World Health Organization (International Histological Classification of Tumours, No. 19)

The histological classification of tumours of the upper respiratory tract and ear, which appears on pages 3–18, contains the morphology code numbers of the International Classification of Diseases for Oncology (ICD-O)[2] and/or the Systematized Nomenclature of Medicine (SNOMED)[3].

The publications in the series *International Histological Classification of Tumours* are not intended to serve as textbooks but rather to promote the adoption of uniform terminology that will facilitate communication among cancer workers. For this reason literature references have been omitted and readers are referred to standard works for bibliographies.

Acknowledgements

The photomicrographs reproduced in this volume were taken by Mr. Tan Tee Chok, Department of Pathology, National University of Singapore. The costs of colour reproduction were borne by donations from the Lee Foundation of Singapore and the Singapore Cancer Society.

---

[2] World Health Organization (1990) International Classification of Diseases for Oncology. Geneva
[3] College of American Pathologists (1982) Systematized Nomenclature of Medicine. Chicago

Contents

Introduction

This volume deals with tumours occurring in the following sites:

Nasal cavity and paranasal sinuses
Nasopharynx
Larynx, hypopharynx and trachea
External ear
Middle and inner ear

The classification of tumours arising from each of the anatomical sites listed above is given separately. However, since the same tumour type may occur in more than one site, the definitions and illustrations have been grouped together. The classification is based on the histological characteristics of the tumours and is therefore concerned with morphologically identifiable cell types and histological patterns as seen with conventional light microscopy. Although many of the histological terms and definitions have histogenetic implications, this classification is not primarily based on histogenesis.

The term "tumour" is used synonymously with neoplasm. The term "tumour-like" is applied to non-neoplastic lesions which clinically or morphologically resemble neoplasms; they are included in this classification because of their importance in differential diagnosis. The terminology adopted for individual tumours is based on their general acceptance and world-wide usage. Synonyms are included only if they have been widely used in the literature or if they are considered helpful in understanding the lesions. In such cases the preferred terms are given first followed by the synonyms within parentheses.

Grading of tumours of the same histological type is performed to provide some indication of their aggressiveness, which may relate in turn to prognosis or treatment. Here, one considers the degree of cytological and architectural similarity to the presumed tissue of origin, as well as nuclear pleomorphism and mitotic activity. Four categories may be distinguished:

Grade 1. Well differentiated: a tumour with histological and cellular features that closely resemble the presumed tissue of origin

Grade 2. Moderately differentiated: a tumour with histological features intermediate between well differentiated and poorly differentiated

Grade 3. Poorly differentiated: a tumour with histological and cellular features which only barely resemble the presumed tissue of origin

Grade 4. Undifferentiated or anaplastic: a tumour with no resemblance to the presumed tissue of origin

Well- and moderately differentiated tumours can be grouped together as low grade, and poorly differentiated and undifferentiated as high grade. When a tumour shows different grades of differentiation, the higher grade should determine the final categorization. Tumour behaviour and prognosis are also influenced by factors other than histological grade. Special consideration should be given to the patterns of growth and spread of the tumour and the stage or extent of tumour at the time of diagnosis. The resectability of the tumour, involvement of cranial bones, interference with respiration and secondary infection are also important considerations in tumours of the upper respiratory tract.

Histological Classification of Tumours of the Upper Respiratory Tract and Ear

Nasal Cavity and Paranasal Sinuses (Excluding Nasal Vestibule)

1   **Epithelial Tumours**

1.1   *Benign*
1.1.1   Sinonasal papilloma (4)[a] . . . . 8121/0[b]
1.1.1.1 Exophytic papilloma (4.1) 8121/0
1.1.1.2 Inverted papilloma (4.2) 8121/1
1.1.1.3 Columnar cell papilloma (4.3) 8121/1
1.1.2   Pleomorphic adenoma (7) 8940/0
1.1.3   Myoepithelioma (8) 8982/0
1.1.4   Oncocytoma (9) 8290/0
1.1.5   Basal cell (basaloid) adenoma (10) 8147/0

1.2   *Malignant*
1.2.1   Sinonasal carcinoma (26) 8121/3
1.2.1.1 Squamous cell carcinoma (26.1) 8070/3
1.2.1.2 Cylindrical cell carcinoma (26.2) 8121/3
1.2.2   Verrucous squamous cell carcinoma (22) 8051/3
1.2.3   Spindle cell carcinoma (23) 8074/3
1.2.4   Adenocarcinoma (28) 8140/3
1.2.5   Papillary adenocarcinoma (29) 8260/3
1.2.6   Intestinal-type adenocarcinoma (30) 8144/3
1.2.7   Acinic cell carcinoma (31) 8550/3

---

[a] The numbers in parentheses refer to items in the definitions and explanatory notes.
[b] Morphology codes of International Classification of Diseases for Oncology (ICD-O) and/or Systematized Nomenclature of Medicine (SNOMED).

2   Soft Tissue Tumours

3   Tumours of Bone and Cartilage

3.1   *Benign*
3.1.1   Chondroma (70) 9220/0
3.1.2   Osteoma (72) 9180/0
3.1.3   Osteoid osteoma (73) 9191/0
3.1.4   Osteoblastoma (74) 9200/0
3.1.5   Ossifying fibroma (75) 9262/0
3.1.6   Giant cell tumour (76) 9250/1

3.2   *Malignant*
3.2.1   Chondrosarcoma (77) 9220/3
3.2.2   Osteosarcoma (78) 9180/3
3.2.3   Malignant giant cell tumour (76) 9250/3
3.2.4   Ewing sarcoma (79) 9260/3

4   Malignant Lymphomas (80)   9590/3

4.1   Non-Hodgkin lymphoma (conventional types) (81)   9591/3
4.2   Extramedullary plasmacytoma (82) 9731/3
4.3   Midline malignant reticulosis (83) 9702/3
4.4   Histiocytic lymphoma (84) 9723/3
4.5   Hodgkin disease (85) 9650/3

5   Miscellaneous Tumours

5.1   *Benign*
5.1.1   Meningioma (87) 9530/0
5.1.2   Ameloblastoma (88) 9310/0
5.1.3   Melanotic neuroectodermal tumour (89) 9363/0
5.1.4   Mature teratoma (91) 9080/0

5.2   *Malignant*
5.2.1   Malignant melanoma (92) 8720/3
5.2.2   Olfactory neuroblastoma (93) 9522/3
5.2.3   Chordoma (94) 9370/3
5.2.4   Malignant germ cell tumours (95)

Nasopharynx

Larynx, Hypopharynx and Trachea

1   Epithelial Tumours and Precancerous Lesions

1.1   *Benign*
1.1.1   Papilloma (6) 8052/0
         Papillomatosis (6) 8060/0
1.1.2   Pleomorphic adenoma (7) 8940/0
1.1.3   Basal cell (basaloid) adenoma (10) 8140/0

1.2   *Dysplasia and Carcinoma In Situ*
1.2.1   Squamous cell dysplasia (18)   74009
1.2.1.1 Mild dysplasia (18.1)   74006
1.2.1.2 Moderate dysplasia (18.2)   74007
1.2.1.3 Severe dysplasia (18.3)   74008
1.2.2   Carcinoma in situ (19) 8070/2

1.3   *Malignant*
1.3.1   Squamous cell carcinoma (21) 8070/3
1.3.2   Verrucous squamous cell carcinoma (22) 8051/3
1.3.3   Spindle cell carcinoma (23) 8074/3
1.3.4   Adenoid squamous cell carcinoma (24) 8075/3
1.3.5   Basaloid squamous cell carcinoma (25) 8094/3
1.3.6   Adenocarcinoma (28) 8140/3
1.3.7   Acinic cell carcinoma (31) 8550/3
1.3.8   Mucoepidermoid carcinoma (32) 8430/3
1.3.9   Adenoid cystic carcinoma (33) 8200/3
1.3.10   Carcinoma in pleomorphic adenoma (35) 8941/3
1.3.11   Epithelial-myoepithelial carcinoma (36) 8562/3
1.3.12   Clear cell carcinoma (37) 8310/3
1.3.13   Adenosquamous carcinoma (38) 8560/3
1.3.14   Giant cell carcinoma (39) 8031/3
1.3.15   Salivary duct carcinoma (40) 8500/3
1.3.16   Carcinoid tumour (41) 8240/3
1.3.17   Atypical carcinoid tumour (42) 8246/3
1.3.18   Small cell carcinoma (43) 8041/3
1.3.19   Lymphoepithelial carcinoma (44) 8082/3

External Ear (Pinna and External Auditory Meatus)

1   **Epithelial Tumours and Precancerous Lesions**

1.1   *Benign*
1.1.1   Squamous cell papilloma (1) 8052/0
1.1.2   Trichoepithelioma (2) 8100/0
1.1.3   Pilomatrixoma (3) 8110/0
1.1.4   Pleomorphic adenoma (7) 8940/0
1.1.5   Ceruminous adenoma (12) 8420/0
1.1.6   Syringocystadenoma papilliferum (13) 8406/0
1.1.7   Sebaceous adenoma (14) 8410/0

1.2   *Dysplasia*
1.2.1   Solar keratosis (17)   72850

1.3   *Malignant*
1.3.1   Basal cell carcinoma (20) 8090/3
1.3.2   Squamous cell carcinoma (21) 8070/3
1.3.3   Verrucous squamous cell carcinoma (22) 8051/3
1.3.4   Spindle cell carcinoma (23) 8074/3
1.3.5   Adenoid squamous cell carcinoma (24) 8075/3
1.3.6   Ceruminous adenocarcinoma (12) 8420/3
1.3.7   Sebaceous carcinoma (14) 8410/3
1.3.8   Adenocarcinoma (28) 8140/3
1.3.9   Mucoepidermoid carcinoma (32) 8430/3
1.3.10   Adenoid cystic carcinoma (33) 8200/3

2   **Soft Tissue Tumours**

2.1   *Benign*
2.1.1   Aggressive fibromatosis (46) 8821/1
2.1.2   Fibrous histiocytoma (49) 8830/0
2.1.3   Leiomyoma (51) 8890/0
2.1.4   Haemangioma (53) 9120/0
2.1.5   Neurilemmoma (56) 9560/0
2.1.6   Neurofibroma (57) 9540/0

8   Tumour-like Lesions

Middle and Inner Ear

1   **Epithelial Tumours**

1.1   *Benign*
1.1.1   Adenoma of middle ear (15) 8140/0
1.1.2   Papillary adenoma (16) 8260/0

1.2   *Malignant*
1.2.1   Squamous cell carcinoma (21) 8070/3
1.2.2   Verrucous squamous cell carcinoma (22) 8051/3
1.2.3   Adenocarcinoma of middle ear (15) 8140/3
1.2.4   Papillary adenocarcinoma (16) 8260/3
1.2.5   Carcinoid tumour (41) 8240/3

2   **Soft Tissue Tumours**

2.1   *Benign*
2.1.1   Myxoma (48) 8840/0
2.1.2   Lipoma (50) 8850/0
2.1.3   Haemangioma (53) 9120/0
2.1.4   Neurilemmoma (56) 9560/0
2.1.5   Neurofibroma (57) 9540/0
2.1.6   Paraganglioma (59) 8693/1

2.2   *Malignant*
2.2.1   Rhabdomyosarcoma (63) 8900/3
2.2.2   Malignant nerve sheath tumour (66) 9560/3
2.2.3   Malignant paraganglioma (59) 8693/3
2.2.4   Synovial sarcoma (68) 9040/3

3   **Tumours of Bone and Cartilage**

3.1   *Benign*
3.1.1   Chondroblastoma (71) 9230/0
3.1.2   Osteoma (72) 9180/0
3.1.3   Giant cell tumour (76) 9250/1

3.2   *Malignant*
3.2.1   Chondrosarcoma (77) 9220/3
3.2.2   Osteosarcoma (78) 9180/3

Definitions and Explanatory Notes

Epithelial Tumours and Precancerous Lesions

1 Squamous Cell Papilloma (Fig. 1)

A benign epithelial neoplasm formed of stratified squamous epithelium.

The tumour is exophytic and consists of a thickened layer of well-differentiated stratified squamous epithelium covering arborescent stalks of fibrovascular stroma. Intercellular bridges and/or varying degrees of keratinization are present.

2 Trichoepithelioma

A benign skin tumour with hair follicle differentiation.

The tumour consists of basaloid cells arranged in compact masses or lace-like networks around keratin-filled microcysts. It has a prominent fibrous stromal component which typically projects into the epithelial elements simulating abortive hair follicles. The tumour is non-ulcerative and may be pigmented. It is often multiple.

3 Pilomatrixoma (Fig. 2)

This tumour usually occurs as a fairly well-defined subepidermal mass. It consists of deeply basophilic masses of small basaloid cells which merge, often abruptly, with pale eosinophilic masses of necrotic epithelium with non-staining nuclei ("ghost" cells). Also present are areas of calcification, cell debris and keratin associated with a foreign-body giant cell reaction.

4 Sinonasal Papilloma (Schneiderian Papilloma)

A benign epithelial tumour of the sinonasal tract composed of well-differentiated columnar or ciliated respiratory epithelium with variable squamous differentiation.

These tumours are generally polypoid and unilateral and comprise three histopathological types (see below).

4.1 Exophytic Papilloma (Fungiform Papilloma) (Figs. 3, 4)

This is a warty tumour occurring almost exclusively on the nasal septum. It is composed of papillary fronds covered by stratified squamous epithelium that is frequently admixed with respiratory epithelium and contains scattered mucin-secreting cells. Recurrences are common. Malignant transformation is very rare.

4.2 Inverted Papilloma (Figs. 5–7)

This is the most common type of sinonasal papilloma. The tumour occurs almost exclusively in the lateral wall of the nasal cavity and in the paranasal sinuses. It is composed of invaginating crypts, thick ribbons or islands of non-keratinizing squamous epithelium which may alternate with or be covered by pseudostratified columnar (cylindrical) or ciliated respiratory epithelium; the multilayered epithelium typically contains mucous cells and mucin-filled microcysts. The infolding of the mucosa may result in the presence of apparently discontinuous cell masses lying deep to the epithelial surface, but the basement membrane is intact and may be shown to be continuous with that of the surface epithelium. Foci of surface keratinization are occasionally present. A few regular mitoses are present in the parabasal layers and there may be mild nuclear irregularities and hyperchromatism, but there is no gross disturbance of polarity. Inflammatory cells, mainly eosinophils and neutrophils, are present in the loose connective tissue stroma and among the epithelial cells. The tumour grows by extension to involve the contiguous sinonasal epithelium. Recurrences are common. Carcinoma, as shown by stromal invasion, supervenes in some cases. The presence of severe atypia or marked keratinization in an inverted papilloma should arouse suspicion of malignant transformation.

4.3 Columnar Cell Papilloma
(Cylindrical Cell Papilloma, Oncocytic Papilloma) (Figs. 8, 9)

This is the least common type of sinonasal papilloma. It is composed of exophytic fronds and endophytic invaginations lined by pseudo-stratified or multilayered columnar cells with oncocytic features. The cells have uniform hyperchromatic nuclei and abundant eosinophilic, occasionally granular, cytoplasm. Intraepithelial microcysts containing mucin and neutrophil leucocytes are usually present. The tumour resembles inverted papilloma (item 4.2) in its sites of occurrence and clinical behaviour.

5 Nasopharyngeal Papilloma

A benign tumour arising from the surface epithelium of the nasopharynx.

Papillomas of the nasopharynx are exceptionally rare. They may exhibit an exophytic or inverted structure like sinonasal papillomas (item 4).

6 Papilloma/Papillomatosis of the Larynx (Figs. 10–13)

A benign epithelial neoplasm of the larynx formed mainly of stratified squamous epithelium.

The tumours are exophytic and consist mainly of branching papillary fronds of well-differentiated stratified squamous epithelium containing cores of fibrovascular stroma. The tumour may also contain respiratory epithelium with mucous and ciliated cells. The basal layers are often hyperplastic, and mitoses may be present. Laryngeal papillomas tend to recur after removal. A rare form of papillomatosis occurs in which there is progressive involvement of the upper and lower respiratory tracts.

Laryngeal papillomas may be subdivided histologically into a non-keratinizing type and a less common keratinizing type in which the superficial layers show keratinization with orthokeratosis and parakeratosis. *Non-keratinizing papillomas* are often multiple, occur primarily in children and are usually related to human papilloma virus infection. They stubbornly recur but have a low malignant potential unless irradiated. Some tumours may undergo spontaneous involution. *Keratinizing papillomas* are usually solitary, occur mainly in adults, are generally not virus related and have a malignant potential. The presence of epithelial dysplasia in an adult papilloma should be regarded as suspicious of malignancy.

7 Pleomorphic Adenoma (Mixed Tumour) (Fig. 14)

A tumour of pleomorphic structure containing luminal-type ductal epithelial cells, myoepithelial cells and tissues of mucoid, myxoid or chondroid appearance.

The tumour contains trabecular, tubular and/or cystic structures which are lined by cuboidal or columnar ductal epithelium and surrounded by irregular sheaths or masses of modified myoepithelial cells which tend to fade off into the stroma. Nests of keratinizing squamous cells may be present, and there may be foci of cylindromatous structure. Mitoses are absent or rare. The stroma is fibrous and focally exhibits mucoid, myxoid or chondroid features; there may be foci of calcification or ossification. Epithelial mucin (PAS- and mucicarmine-positive) may be present in the duct lumina and connective tissue-type mucin (alcian blue-positive) in the mucomyxoid and chondroid areas. Biopsy samples with a predominant cylindromatous component may be mistaken for adenoid cystic carcinoma and those containing mucin-secreting cells and squamous cells for mucoepidermoid carcinoma. The diagnosis of pleomorphic adenoma rests on the demonstration of the characteristic epithelial, myoepithelial and mucomyxoid or chondroid elements. The tumour is usually well demarcated but may recur after removal. Malignant change is rare.

8 Myoepithelioma (Myoepithelial Adenoma) and Malignant Myoepithelioma (Myoepithelial Carcinoma) (Fig. 15)

Tumours composed of myoepithelial cells without a ductal epithelial component.

The tumours are composed of spindle-shaped cells with finely granular cytoplasm, clear cells with eccentric nuclei, polygonal cells with hyaline cytoplasm (plasmacytoid or hyaline cells) or mixtures of these cell types. The cells may be arranged in compact sheets and fascicles or in loose myxoid or reticular patterns. The tumour cells are usually immunoreactive for cytokeratin, myosin, muscle-specific actin and S-100 protein. Ultrastructurally they have myofilaments, basement membranes and desmosomes.

Myoepithelial tumours are usually benign but tend to grow more aggressively than pleomorphic adenoma (item 7). The myoepithelioma is usually encapsulated and is distinguished from pleomorphic adenoma, of which it may be a variant, by the lack of a ductal epithelial component. Malignant myoepithelioma is characterized by infiltrative growth, cytologic atypia, increased mitotic activity and a tendency to metastasize. It appears probable that some clear cell carcinomas (item 37) may actually represent malignant clear cell myoepithelioma.

9 Oncocytoma (Figs. 16, 17)

An epithelial tumour composed of large columnar or polyhedral cells with centrally placed vesicular or hyperchromatic nuclei and abundant, intensely eosinophilic granular cytoplasm.

The tumour cells may be arranged in compact sheets and cords or in tubular or papillary structures. Their cytoplasmic eosinophilia may vary in intensity, and many tumours contain a mixture of pale and dark cells. The cells stain positively with PTAH or cresyl violet, and electron microscopy reveals a large number of mitochondria. The tumour is well demarcated and may be partially encapsulated. Mitoses are rare. The distinction between oncocytoma and oncocytic metaplasia (item 124) is often difficult; the latter occurs far more frequently in the upper respiratory tract.

10 Basal Cell (Basaloid) Adenoma (Figs. 18–20)

A tumour of salivary gland type composed mainly of small uniform basaloid cells and not having a mucoid or chondroid component as in pleomorphic adenoma.

The tumours exhibits a variety of growth patterns: a *tubular* variant in which the basaloid cells are found on the outer aspect of narrow anastomosing ductal structures lined by luminal type cells, a *trabecular* variant in which the basaloid cells are arranged in anastomosing cords which may have a centrally placed component of larger or paler cells, a *solid* variant in which the basaloid cells are arranged in compact masses with a palisaded outer layer and, very rarely, a *membranous* variant (dermal analogue type) in which the cell masses have palisaded outer layers and prominent hyaline basement membranes. The tumours are encapsulated or well circumscribed, have bland cytologic features and, with the exception of the membranous variety have limited tendency to recur after removal. The basal cell adenoma is rare in the upper respiratory tract and should be distinguished from well-differentiated adenocarcinoma (item 28); the latter tumour may have an equally bland histomorphology but is infiltrative.

11 Ectopic Pituitary Adenoma (Fig. 21)

A benign tumour composed of anterior pituitary-type cells occurring in the wall of the nasopharynx or nasal cavity.

The tumour cells are typically of the chromophobe variety and may be arranged in sheets, columns or nests separated by thin-walled vessels or bands of connective tissue. The diagnosis is confirmed by immunocytologic demonstration of chromogranin and various pituitary hormones. Immunostaining generally reveals a predominance of one cell type. The tumour is associated with a clinically apparent hormonal disorder and/or a clinically detectable mass. The sellar pituitary appears normal. The tumour is rare and probably arises from anterior pituitary-type cells occurring in the wall of the nasopharynx, nasal cavity or the sphenoid sinus. It should be distinguished from heterotopic pituitary tissue (item 102.4) and from adenomas of the sellar pituitary that have extended downwards through the sphenoid bone.

12 Ceruminous Adenoma and Adenocarcinoma (Figs. 22–24)

Tumours of ceruminous glands.

Ceruminous tumours are similar to other apocrine gland tumours and show the same range of structural variation. The ceruminous adenoma generally consists of lobules of bilayered glands separated by fibrous, occasionally hyalinized stroma. The inner layer is composed of cuboidal or columnar epithelial cells with eosinophilic cytoplasm and apical snouts; the cytoplasm may contain haemosiderin granules or ceroid pigment. The outer layer is composed of myoepithelial cells. The glandular structures may contain mucoid material. They often vary considerably in size and may exhibit papillary projections; back-to-back patterns are common. The distinction between ceruminous adenoma and adenocarcinoma may be difficult on histologic grounds. Ceruminous adenocarcinoma is generally not bilayered and exhibits infiltrative growth, increased mitotic activity and mild to moderate cytologic atypia.

Other glandular neoplasms occurring in the external auditory meatus, namely pleomorphic adenoma, syringocystadenoma papilliferum, adenoid cystic carcinoma and mucoepidermoid carcinoma, may also arise from ceruminous glands.

13 Syringocystadenoma Papilliferum

A papillary-cystic tumour with apocrine differentiation.

The tumour consists of intercommunicating cystic spaces and papillary projections lined mainly by bilayered epithelium comprising an inner layer of columnar cells with apocrine-type decapitation secretion and an outer or basal layer of cuboidal or fusiform cells with myoepithelial features. The cystic spaces often appear as invaginations of the surface epithelium.

14 Sebaceous Adenoma and Sebaceous Carcinoma

Epithelial tumours with sebaceous differentiation.

Sebaceous adenoma is a well-circumscribed tumour consisting of lobules of mature sebaceous cells with peripheral zones of basaloid-type germinative epithelium. *Sebaceous carcinoma* is an infiltrative tumour composed of sheets of predominantly undifferentiated cells with cytologic atypia, increased mitotic activity and scattered foci of sebaceous differentiation.

15 Adenoma and Adenocarcinoma of the Middle Ear (Fig. 25)

Epithelial tumours of glandular morphology occurring in the middle ear.

These tumours probably originate from middle ear mucosa. They are usually non-encapsulated and are composed of small, closely packed glands with a tendency for back-to-back arrangement. The glands are lined by a single layer of fairly uniform cuboidal or low columnar epithelium with rounded hyperchromatic nuclei, eosinophilic cytoplasm and well-defined cell margins. Intraluminal mucin may be present. There is no myoepithelial component. Compact sheets or cords of tumour cells may be present. Mitoses are rare. The middle ear adenoma is slow-growing and non-destructive. Tumours with locally invasive destructive growth are classified as adenocarcinoma although metastases have not been recorded.

The middle ear adenoma may contain cells with argyrophil (Grimelius – positive) granules and electron dense granules that are typically not membrane bound. It should be distinguished from the carcinoid tumour (item 41) and paraganglioma (item 59). The distinction from carcinoid tumour may be difficult because some middle ear adenomas also contain cells with membrane bound dense-core granules.

16 Papillary Adenoma
and Papillary Adenocarcinoma of the Middle and Inner Ear
(Fig. 26)

These rare tumours are usually found in the temporal bones. They may originate from the mucosa lining the middle ear cleft or from the endolymphatic sac of the inner ear. The tumours have a papillary-cystic structure with vascular stroma covered by cuboidal or low columnar cells with eosinophilic or clear cytoplasm. Mucin stains are generally negative, but gland-like spaces containing mucoid or colloid-like material may be present. The tumours often grow aggressively. Locally infiltrative and destructive tumours may be classified as papillary adenocarcinoma, although metastases have not been recorded.

17 Solar Keratosis (Actinic Keratosis) (Fig. 27)

Epidermal dysplasia due to actinic radiation.
    The epidermis may be hyperplastic or atrophic and shows disorderly maturation with varying degrees of hyperkeratosis, parakeratosis, acantholysis, cytologic atypia and increased mitotic activity. The accumulation of a mass of keratin over the lesion may lead to the formation of a cutaneous "horn". The dermis shows basophilic degeneration of collagen and elastosis. The lesion is precancerous; squamous cell carcinoma develops frequently in untreated cases.

18 Squamous Cell Dysplasia (Figs. 28–30)

A precancerous lesion of squamous epithelium characterized by cellular atypia and loss of normal maturation and stratification short of carcinoma in situ.
    Three grades of dysplasia are recognized on the basis of the degree of nuclear abnormalities and the proportion of epithelial thickness showing loss of normal stratification. Dysplasia may coexist with invasive carcinoma; the potential for developing invasive carcinoma increases with the grade of dysplasia.

18.1 Mild Dysplasia (Fig. 28)

The nuclear abnormalities are slight and are most marked in the basal third of the epithelial thickness. They are minimal in the upper layers where the cells show maturation and stratification. A few mitoses may be present in the parabasal layers; there are no abnormal mitoses. Keratosis and chronic inflammation are usually present. The lesion should be distinguisghed from squamous cell hyperplasia (item 119).

18.2 Moderate Dysplasia (Fig. 29)

The nuclear abnormalities are more marked than in mild dysplasia and nucleoli tend to be prominent. These changes are most marked in the lower two-thirds of the epithelial thickness. Moderate nuclear abnormalities may persist up to the surface, but cell maturation and stratification are evident in the upper layers. Mitoses are present in the parabasal and intermediate layers; there are no abnormal mitoses. The lesion may be associated with keratosis.

18.3 Severe Dysplasia (Fig. 30)

The epithelium shows marked nuclear abnormalities and loss of maturation involving more than two-thirds of the epithelial thickness with some stratification of the most superficial layers. Nuclear pleomorphism is common, and some of the cells may have bizarre nuclei. In some areas the nucleoli are very prominent, but in others all the nuclei are hyperchromatic. Mitoses are present high up in the epithelium, and atypical mitoses may be found. The cells are generally not as crowded as in classic carcinoma in situ and are usually more differentiated with intercellular bridges between the atypical cells. The presence of some maturation and stratification of the cells in the most superficial layers distinguishes the lesion from carcinoma in situ (item 19). The lesion is frequently associated with keratosis. Severe dysplasia has the same high risk for developing invasive carcinoma as carcinoma in situ and is therefore grouped with it for clinical purposes.

19 Carcinoma In Situ (Intraepithelial Carcinoma) (Figs. 31–33)

A lesion in which the full thickness of the squamous epithelium shows the cellular features of carcinoma without stromal invasion.

Laryngeal carcinoma in situ is usually of the large cell keratinizing type with the epithelial cells having markedly abnormal hyperchromatic nuclei and variable cytoplasmic keratinization; there is a close resemblance to severe dysplasia (item 18.3). In some cases the cells have scanty cytoplasm with little or no evidence of squamous differentiation, as in classic carcinoma in situ of the cervix uteri. Mitoses occur high up in the epithelium; atypical mitoses may be present. The lesion may extend into the ducts of adjacent seromucinous glands, but the basement membrane is intact throughout its extent.

The term *papillary carcinoma in situ* (non-invasive papillary carcinoma) is applied to exophytic papillary tumours composed of cores of fibrovascular stroma covered by squamous epithelium with cytological features similar to those in conventional carcinoma in situ. The presence of severe cytologic atypia, increased mitotic activity and loss of normal stratification distinguishes them from the laryngeal papillomas with epithelial dysplasia occurring in adults (item 6).

Laryngeal carcinoma in situ may occur as an isolated lesion or in association with invasive carcinoma; the absence of stromal invasion should therefore be confirmed by sampling the entire biopsy specimen.

20 Basal Cell Carcinoma (Fig. 34)

A locally invasive, slowly growing tumour arising from and usually resembling the basal cells of the epidermis and hair follicles.

The tumour consists of compact masses of uniform cells with attachments to the basal layer of the epidermis or hair follicles. The cell masses usually show palisading of the peripheral layer and may contain cystic spaces or sharply defined foci of squamous differentiation. The stroma surrounding the tumour masses may show mucoid changes. Basal cell carcinoma of the external ear has the same range of histological appearances as those arising elsewhere in the skin but tends to be more aggressive. It may extend into the middle ear or mastoid if inadequately treated.

21 Squamous Cell Carcinoma (Figs. 35, 36)

A malignant epithelial tumour with squamous differentiation characterized by the formation of keratin and/or the presence of intercellular bridges.

Squamous cell carcinomas of the upper respiratory tract manifest the same range of histological appearances as those arising in other sites. The tumours are graded according to the degree of differentiation, cellular pleomorphism and mitotic activity. Well-differentiated carcinomas have a close resemblance to normal squamous epithelium and contain varying proportions of basal-type cells and squamous cells with intercellular bridges and full keratinization; mitoses are scanty. Moderately differentiated carcinomas have less keratinization and more nuclear pleomorphism; there are more mitoses, including abnormal mitoses. Keratinization and intercellular bridges are minimal and barely discernible in poorly differentiated carcinomas. Grading has been found to be of some prognostic value although the assessment of the degree of differentiation is essentially subjective and influenced by variations in sampling. The term *microinvasive squamous cell carcinoma* is used to describe cases in which tumour invasion, occurring as scattered tongues or discrete foci, is confined to the area just below the basement membrane.

The term *papillary squamous cell carcinoma* (invasive papillary carcinoma) is applied to invasive squamous cell carcinomas which have an exophytic papillary component with the histological features of papillary carcinoma in situ (item 19). The invasive component is often inconspicuous and may require serial sections or multiple samples for identification. Such tumours should be distinguished from verrucous squamous cell carcinoma which has bland cytologic features and minimal atypia (item 22).

22 Verrucous Squamous Cell Carcinoma (Figs. 37–39)

A warty variant of squamous cell carcinoma characterized by a predominantly exophytic overgrowth of well-differentiated keratinizing epithelium with locally aggressive pushing margins.

The tumour is usually bulky and presents a warty papillomatous surface. It is usually superficial and tends to compress and erode local structures in the form of bulbous acanthotic folds rather than as insinuating or tentacular infiltrates. The neoplastic epithelial masses may contain microabscesses. Vertical sections of the neoplasm show epithelial spires capped and separated by a thick parakeratotic or keratotic layer. Keratohyaline granules are generally sparse. The stroma surrounding the pushing margins of the tumour is heavily infiltrated by chronic inflammatory cells, and there may be occasional foreign body granulomas induced by keratin. Mitoses are rare, and the tumour cells have bland cytologic features. These papilloma-like appearances and the orderly maturation sequence belie the locally destructive nature of the tumour. Biopsy material from superficial areas may not show the characteristic histological features. The tumour is slow growing and lacks the ability to metastasize. Verrucous carcinoma is distinguished from conventional well-differentiated squamous cell carcinoma and papillary squamous cell carcinoma (item 21) by its minimal atypia, growth pattern and absence of metastasis. Foci of conventional squamous cell carcinoma may coexist with verrucous carcinoma; a full examination of the resected specimen is therefore essential.

23 Spindle Cell Carcinoma (Figs. 40, 41)

A bimorphic carcinoma with a component that is identifiable as a squamous cell carcinoma and an underlying or adjacent spindle cell or pleomorphic cell component.

The tumour component that is identifiable as a squamous cell carcinoma may be in situ or invasive. It is usually inconspicuous and may require examination of multiple blocks of tissue taken from the base, margins and depths of the tumour for identification. The bulk of the tumour resembles a sarcoma and comprises spindled or pleomorphic cells with atypical or bizarre nuclei and abnormal mitoses; multinucleated tumour cells may be present. Some of the tumour cells may contain intracytoplasmic hyaline globules. Most of these tumours are rapidly growing, bulky and polypoid; some are flat, ulcerative or infiltrative. Their biological behaviour resembles conventional squamous cell carcinoma. Opinions have varied on whether the sarcomatoid component is benign or malignant, and whether it is epithelial or mesenchymal in origin. Metastases from the tumour usually contain only epithelial elements and are only rarely sarcomatous. On the basis of its immunohistologic and ultrastructural characteristics the spindle cell/pleomorphic cell component has been variously reported as being of epithelial or mesenchymal origin. It is therefore probable that tumours with these histological features are not homogeneous but comprise: *spindle cell squamous carcinoma* in which the stroma of a squamous cell carcinoma contains malignant spindle or pleomorphic tumour cells that are demonstrably epithelial and derived from the squamous cell component; *squamous cell carcinoma with pseudosarcomatous stroma* in which a squamous cell carcinoma is associated with atypical but nonneoplastic fibroblastic or fibrohistiocytic proliferation; and rare examples of true *carcinosarcoma* in which a sarcoma of fibroblastic, fibrohistiocytic or other soft tissue origin coexists with squamous cell carcinoma.

24 Adenoid Squamous Cell Carcinoma (Fig. 42)

A squamous cell carcinoma in which pseudoglandular spaces or lumina are present.
    The pseudoglandular structure in this variant of squamous cell carcinoma results from acantholysis of the tumour cells. There is no evidence of true glandular differentiation or mucin production. The tumour is generally of low-grade malignancy. It should be distinguished from adenosquamous carcinoma (item 38).

25 Basaloid Squamous Cell Carcinoma (Fig. 43)

A bimorphic carcinoma with mixed basaloid and squamous cell components.
    The basaloid component of this tumour is usually the more prominent and consists of small cells with hyperchromatic nuclei and scanty cytoplasm arranged in compact lobular masses or cords with attachments to the surface epithelium. Cells with larger vesicular nuclei may also be present. The tumour masses exhibit peripheral palisading, cystic or gland-like spaces that may contain mucoid material and focal squamous differentiation. Normal and abnormal mitoses and areas of necrosis are common. The stroma is frequently hyalinized. The component that is identifiable as a squamous cell carcinoma may be in situ or invasive; the presence of this component helps to distinguish the tumour from the solid variety of adenoid cystic carcinoma (item 33). The tumour is highly malignant.

26 Sinonasal Carcinoma (Schneiderian Carcinoma)
(Figs. 44–46)

Carcinomas arising from the respiratory epithelium lining the nasal cavity and sinuses may be subdivided into keratinizing squamous cell carcinoma and cylindrical cell or non-keratinizing carcinoma. Rare variants of squamous cell carcinoma, namely verrucous carcinoma (item 22) and spindle cell carcinoma (item 23), may also arise from the sinonasal epithelium.

26.1 Squamous Cell Carcinoma
(Keratinizing Squamous Cell Carcinoma) (Fig. 44)

This type of sinonasal carcinoma shows squamous differentiation with presence of intercellular bridges and/or keratinization over most of its extent. It may be well, moderately or poorly differentiated.

26.2 Cylindrical Cell Carcinoma (Non-keratinizing Carcinoma, Transitional-type Carcinoma) (Figs. 45, 46)

This type of sinonasal carcinoma is composed of cells of respiratory epithelial type. The tumour is usually polypoid and exophytic with a smooth, corrugated or papillary surface. It is composed of thick ribbons and multilayered masses of cells which often appear as invaginations of the surface epithelium. The overall pattern is usually one of en bloc invasion with a pushing border and focal stroma infiltration. The tumour cells are mainly cylindrical and often set at right angles to the underlying basement membrane. The nuclei are hyperchromatic and atypical and show increased mitotic activity including abnormal mitoses. Squamous metaplasia is common, and when extensive the tumour may be indistinguishable from squamous cell carcinoma (item 26.1). Foci of small cell carcinoma (item 43) and/or high-grade adenocarcinoma (item 28) are occasionally present; a full examination of the resected specimen is therefore essential.

27 Nasopharyngeal Carcinoma (Figs. 47–54)

A malignant tumour of the epithelium lining the surface and crypts of the nasopharynx.

The tumour shows no evidence of mucin production or of glandular differentiation. By electron microscopy it has the characteristics of squamous cell carcinoma with tonofilament bundles and desmosomes. The tumour may be subdivided into two main groups according to whether or not there is clear evidence of squamous differentiation by light microscopy.

27.1 Squamous Cell Carcinoma
(Keratinizing Squamous Cell Carcinoma) (Figs. 47, 48)

This type of nasopharyngeal carcinoma shows squamous differentiation with the presence of intercellular bridges and/or keratinization over most of its extent.

27.2 Non-keratinizing Carcinomas (Figs. 49–54)
This group comprises a differentiated type of non-keratinizing carcinoma and an undifferentiated type. These tumours are generally
more radiosensitive than squamous cell carcinoma (item 27.1) and
have stronger relationships with the Epstein-Barr virus. The tumours are often infiltrated by lymphocytes. The term *lymphoepithelial carcinoma* (lymphoepithelioma) is used to describe non-keratinizing carcinomas in which numerous lymphocytes are found among
the tumour cells; the lymphoid elements in such tumours are not
neoplastic.

27.2.1 Differentiated Non-keratinizing Carcinoma (Figs. 49, 50) The
tumour cells show differentiation with a maturation sequence that
results in cells in which squamous differentiation is not evident on
light microscopy. The cells have fairly well-defined cell margins and
show an arrangement that is stratified or pavemented and not syncytial. A plexiform pattern is common.

**27.2.2 Undifferentiated Carcinoma (Undifferentiated Carcinoma of
Nasopharyngeal Type)** (Figs. 51–54) The tumour cells have oval or
round vesicular nuclei and prominent nucleoli. The cell margins are
indistinct, and the tumour exhibits a syncytial rather than pavemented appearance. Spindle-shaped tumour cells, some with
hyperchromatic nuclei, may be present. The tumour cells are arranged in irregular or moderately well-defined masses and/or as
loosely connected cells in a lymphoid stroma. These cytological and
histological features are fairly characteristic and when present in
metastatic tumours, which are particularly common in the upper cer-
vical lymph nodes, may enable a presumptive diagnosis of naopha-
ryngeal carcinoma to be made. Undifferentiated nasopharyngeal
carcinoma may resemble the large cell (centroblastic) or immunoblastic types of malignant lymphoma and may be distinguished from
them by the cohesiveness of the tumour cells and by their positive
immunoreactivity for keratin and negative reaction for the leucocyte
common antigen.

28 Adenocarcinoma (Figs. 55–58)

A malignant epithelial tumour of glandular structure.
    Adenocarcinomas may occur in any part of the upper respiratory
tract but are relatively more common in the ethmoid sinus and the

upper part of the nasal cavity. They may arise from the surface epithelium or from seromucous glands. Their structure may be trabecular, tubular, acinar, microcystic or papillary.

Low-grade adenocarcinomas are composed of glandular or papillary structures lined by a single layer of cuboidal or columnar cells with uniform round or oval nuclei, inconspicuous nucleoli and minimal cytologic atypia. The glandular elements are often packed closely; back-to-back patterns are common. Mitoses are scarce. Calcospherites may be present. The tumours may resemble adenoma or columnar cell papilloma closely but are locally infiltrative and have a higher frequency of local recurrence. *High-grade adenocarcinomas* are composed of irregular glandular structures, trabeculae or solid sheets of cells with nuclear atypia, pleomorphism and high mitotic activity.

29 Papillary Adenocarcinoma (Fig. 59)

The papillary adenocarcinoma occurring in the sinonasal tract and nasopharynx is composed of complex papillary fronds and closely packed glandular structures lined by columnar or pseudostratified cells with vesicular nuclei and eosinophilic cytoplasm. Mucin is present in the cytoplasm and glandular lumina. The tumour is typically continuous with and probably arises from the surface epithelium. Mitoses are uncommon. The tumour is of low-grade malignancy.

30 Intestinal-type (Colonic-type, Mucinous) Adenocarcinoma (Figs. 60, 61)

A tumour with histological features resembling colorectal adenocarcinoma.

The tumour is composed of columnar mucin-secreting cells and goblet cells and has a structure that may be predominantly papillary, glandular, compact or mucinous. Some tumours may contain argentaffin cells and Paneth cells. In the *mucinous adenocarcinoma* a substantial part of the tumour (more than 50%) is occupied by dilated mucin-filled glands lined by columnar mucin-secreting epithelium, lakes of mucin containing fragmented epithelial elements or mucin-filled tumour cells with signet-ring morphology. Cytologic atypia, high mitotic activity and areas of necrosis are common features in all tumours. The tumour grows aggressively and has a poor prognosis. The possibility of metastasis from gastrointestinal adenocarcinoma should be excluded clinically before a tumour is placed in this category.

31 Acinic Cell Carcinoma (Fig. 62)

A tumour composed mainly of cells resembling the serous cells of salivary glands.

The tumour has solid, microcystic, papillary-cystic or follicular growth patterns. It is composed of polyhedral or wedge-shaped cells that typically have small basally placed hyperchromatic nuclei and abundant cytoplasm containing basophil diastase-resistant PAS-positive granules. Clear or vacuolated cells are common; some non-specific glandular cells and a few mucin-secreting cells are occasionally present. The cells characteristically contain amylase. The stroma is scanty and may be hyalinized. Laminated calcified spherules may be present in the stroma and among the tumour cells. The cytological features are bland, and the tumour is of low-grade malignancy with slow infiltrative growth and infrequent metastases.

32 Mucoepidermoid Carcinoma (Figs. 63–65)

A tumour composed of a mixture of squamous cells, mucin-secreting cells and cells of intermediate type.

The ratio of squamous cells to mucin-secreting cells varies, but both cell types should be demonstrable in any tumour that is placed in this category. These cell types are intimately admixed within the tumour. Usually present are ductal structures or cysts lined by mucin-secreting cells alternating with multilayered squamous cells and cells of intermediate type. Mucin-filled cysts are common. The epidermoid component also occurs in the form of compact masses or strands; the squamous cells often have recognizable intercellular bridges, but well-developed keratinization is uncommon. The intermediate-type cells have hyperchromatic nuclei and scanty cytoplasm. Cells with clear or glassy PAS-negative cytoplasm may also be present. The stroma does not have myxoid or chondroid features.

Low-grade mucoepidermoid carcinomas are composed of glandular structures and microcysts which are mainly lined by well-differentiated mucin-secreting cells with foci of intermediate cells and stratified squamous cells of bland appearance. Mitoses are absent or very rare. *High-grade* mucoepidermoid carcinomas are composed mainly of squamous cells and intermediate cells arranged in compact nests and islands; mucin-secreting cells are present but may be scarce. Nuclear pleomorphism is present, and there are frequent mitoses. The tumour should be distinguished from adenosquamous carcinoma (item 38).

33 Adenoid Cystic Carcinoma (Figs. 66–70)

A tumour composed mainly of small uniform basaloid cells forming tubules, cords and/or compact masses that are surrounded and intersected by cylinders of hyaline or mucoid material typically giving a cribriform or lace-like pattern.

This is the most common malignant glandular tumour of the upper respiratory tract. The basaloid tumour cells are uniformly small and have deeply staining nuclei and scanty indistinct cytoplasm. Small ductal-type epithelial cells with vesicular nuclei, eosinophilic cytoplasm and well-defined cell margins may also be present. The cell masses typically contain numerous sharply defined cylindrical spaces containing pale hyaline or mucoid material giving a characteristic cribriform pseudocystic appearance. The tumour cells may also be arranged in tubular or trabecular formations and compact masses which are characteristically ensheathed by pale hyaline zones. The mucohyaline material within the pseudocystic spaces and surrounding the cell masses, mainly proteoglycans and basement membrane-like material, is hyaluronidase sensitive Alcian blue positive and weakly PAS positive after diastase digestion. The tubular spaces lined by ductal epithelium found in some tumours may contain mucin that is diastase resistant PAS positive and mucicarmine positive. Mitoses are generally scarce. The tumour is slow growing but is markedly infiltrative and has a special tendency to grow along nerves. Tumours with a predominantly compact growth pattern are generally associated with more frequent metastases and poorer prognosis.

34 Polymorphous Low-Grade Adenocarcinoma (Terminal Duct Adenocarcinoma)

An infiltrating tumour of minor salivary glands composed of small isomorphic epithelial cells with bland cytologic features and a polymorphous growth pattern.

The tumour occurs almost exclusively in the oral cavity; only a few cases have been documented in the upper respiratory tract. It is composed of small cuboidal cells with uniform ovoid nuclei with finely dispersed chromatin, inconspicuous nucleoli and scanty cytoplasm. The cytologic features are bland, and mitoses are scarce. A variety of structural patterns are evident: solid nests, tubules, anastomosing cords, single-file infiltrates, papillary-cystic structures and cribriform nests. In some cases the tumour cells are arranged concentrically around cell nests, blood vessels or nerves. The tumour has a tendency for perineural infiltration. The stroma is fibrous and may be hyalinized. The tumour is distinguished from adenoid cystic carcinoma (item 33) by the lack of the deeply staining basaloid cells characteristic of the latter neoplasm. The tumour is of low-grade malignancy; it may recur locally and rarely spread to lymph nodes but has little tendency for distant metastases.

35 Carcinoma in Pleomorphic Adenoma

A carcinoma arising in a pleomorphic adenoma.

This tumour has a component identifiable as pleomorphic adenoma (item 7) and a malignant component with features of adenocarcinoma, any of the specific types of salivary gland carcinoma or undifferentiated carcinoma. Only the carcinomatous elements of the tumour are present in metastases. Rare cases in which the tumour and/or its metastases contain carcinomatous and sarcomatous elements are classified as *carcinosarcoma* (malignant mixed tumour).

36 Epithelial-Myoepithelial Carcinoma (Intercalated Duct Carcinoma) (Fig. 71)

A malignant tumour composed of tubules lined by an inner layer of cuboidal or low columnar epithelial cells and outer layers of myoepithelial cells.

The myoepithelial cells are frequently multilayered and have well-defined cell margins and abundant clear cytoplasm containing varying amounts of glycogen. The tubular lumina may contain diastase-resistant, PAS-positive material. The myoepithelial component is generally the more prominent; the ductal-type epithelial component may be inconspicuous in some tumours. Mitoses are rare. The epithelial-myoepithelial units are often closely packed and separated by basement membrane-like material. Microcysts and papillary processes lined by both types of cells may be present. By immunostaining the ductal epithelial cells are reactive for cytokeratin and the myoepithelial cells for S-100 protein and myosin. The tumour may appear well circumscribed but is infiltrative and may be multinodular. Recurrences are common but metastases are rare.

37 Clear Cell Carcinoma (Figs. 72, 73)

A malignant epithelial tumour composed of cells with clear cytoplasm.

The tumour is composed of polygonal cells with vesicular nuclei and abundant vacuolated or water-clear cytoplasm that usually contains glycogen and stains negatively for mucin. Bizarre multinucleated cells may be present. The tumour cells may be arranged in sheets, irregular clusters or glandular formations intersected by fibrous stroma. There is no evidence of squamous differentiation. The tumour should be distinguished from other tumours with areas of clear cell morphology, namely mucoepidermoid carcinoma (item 32), acinic cell carcinoma (item 31), epithelial-myoepithelial carcinoma (item 36), malignant myoepithelioma (item 8) and some soft tissue tumours. The possibility of metastasis from clear cell carcinoma of the kidney or other organs should be excluded clinically before a tumour is placed in this category.

38 Adenosquamous Carcinoma

A malignant tumour with histological features of both adenocarcinoma and squamous cell carcinoma.

This tumour may arise from the ducts of minor salivary or seromucous glands or from the overlying surface epithelium. The component identified as squamous cell carcinoma may be in situ or invasive, and the adenocarcinomatous component comprises glandular structures lined by basaloid, columnar or mucin-secreting cells. The glandular and squamous components occur in close proximity but are generally distinct, unlike mucoepidermoid carcinoma (item 32) in which the squamous and mucin-secreting cells are intimately admixed within individual glandular units or cystic structures. However, the distinction between adenosquamous carcinoma and high-grade mucoepidermoid carcinoma may be difficult. The tumour should also be distinguished from adenoid squamous cell carcinoma (item 24). Adenosquamous carcinoma is a highly malignant tumour with aggressive growth and frequent metastases.

39 Giant Cell Carcinoma

An undifferentiated carcinoma containing many bizarre multinucleated cells.

The tumour cells have abundant eosinophilic cytoplasm which may contain neutrophil leucocytes or cell debris. There is no evidence of squamous or glandular differentiation by light microscopy. This category corresponds with the giant cell carcinoma of lung. It should be distinguished from pleomorphic variants of adenocarcinoma, spindle cell carcinoma (item 23), rhabdomyosarcoma and malignant fibrous histiocytoma.

40 Salivary Duct Carcinoma

This tumour exhibits fairly well-circumscribed islands of tumour cells resembling distended ducts with papillary, cribriform or compact structure and often associated with comedo-type necrosis. Also present are stromal infiltrates that are usually associated with a desmoplastic reaction. The overall structure is reminiscent of ductal carcinoma of breast. The tumour usually grows aggressively and is associated with poor prognosis.

41 Carcinoid Tumour (Typical Carcinoid Tumour) (Fig. 74)

An epithelial tumour of low-grade malignancy composed of bland isomorphic spheroidal cells with histologic, immunocytologic and ultrastructural evidence of neuroendocrine differentiation.

The tumour is composed of ribbons, festoons or compact islands of uniform small cells separated by fibrovascular stroma that may be hyalinized. Tubular or rosette-like structures may be present. The tumour cells have regular round or oval centrally placed nuclei and granular eosinophilic cytoplasm. In some tumours the cells exhibit oncocytic features. There is no necrosis, and mitoses are scarce. Tumours with necrosis, increased mitotic activity and/or nuclear pleomorphism are classified as atypical carcinoid tumours (item 42). Argyrophil granules are demonstrable in the tumour cells by the Grimelius staining technique and membrane-bound, dense-core granules by electron microscopy. By immunostaining the cells typically express cytokeratin, epithelial membrane antigen, chromogranin, neuron-specific enolase and various peptide hormones. The tumour is slow growing. The typical carcinoid tumour occurs but rarely in the upper respiratory tract.

42 Atypical Carcinoid Tumour (Figs. 75, 76)

A carcinoid tumour showing increased mitotic activity and nuclear atypia.

The tumour cells are arranged in nests, ribbons and glandular structures and exhibit nuclear atypia and numerous mitoses. Necrosis is common. The cells are moderately pleomorphic with variable eosinophilic cytoplasm that may contain argyrophil granules. Intraluminal mucin is occasionally present. Dense-core granules are usually demonstrable. The tumour cells usually express positive immunocytologic reactions for cytokeratin and epithelial membrane antigen; positive reactions for neuron-specific enolase, chromogranin and various peptide hormones are often present, but their expression is variable. The tumour is invasive and has a metastatic potential. Atypical carcinoid tumours of the larynx may be immunoreactive for calcitonin and resemble medullary carcinoma of thyroid but show more nuclear atypia and mitotic activity; the possibility of a primary thyroid tumour should be excluded clinically.

43 Small Cell Carcinoma
(Small Cell Neuroendocrine Carcinoma) (Fig. 77)

A highly malignant epithelial tumour composed of small cells with histologic features similar to small cell carcinoma of lung.

The tumour is composed of sheets of small cells with scanty cytoplasm and oval hyperchromatic nuclei with evenly distributed chromatin and inconspicuous nucleoli. The cells may be arranged in insular masses, nests or anastomosing ribbons separated by fibrovascular stroma; rosette-like patterns may also be present. The tumour is histologically indistinguishable from small cell carcinoma of the lung and, like the latter neoplasm, includes an *oat cell* type composed of uniform small cells with barely discernible cytoplasm, an *intermediate cell* type composed of cells with more abundant cytoplasm and a *combined cell* type in which a small cell carcinoma with oat cell and/or intermediate cell morphology has a component of squamous cell carcinoma or adenocarcinoma. Mitoses are numerous, and necrotic changes are common. The tumour cells usually express low molecular weight cytokeratin, epithelial membrane antigen and neuron-specific enolase; positive staining for chromogranin is rare. There is variable neuroendocrine differentiation; argyrophil and dense-core granules are occasionally present but are generally sparse. The tumour is markedly invasive and has a high grade of malignancy. The histological features may resemble those of other small cell tumours, namely some types of lymphoma, embryonal rhabdomyosarcoma, neuroblastoma and Ewing sarcoma; the use of immunocytologic techniques and electron microscopy are helpful in differential diagnosis.

44 Lymphoepithelial Carcinoma (Undifferentiated Carcinoma with Lymphocytic Stroma)

This category refers to carcinomas that are histologically indistinguishable from the "lymphoepithelial carcinoma" of the nasopharynx (item 27.2). The possibility of direct spread or metastasis from a nasopharyngeal primary should be excluded before a tumour is categorized as a primary in other sites.

Soft Tissue Tumours

45 Fibroma

A benign tumour composed exclusively of mature fibroblasts and collagen.

True fibromas are exceptionally rare. Fibrous lesions in the upper respiratory tract usually represent post-inflammatory or reactive fibroblastic proliferations.

46 Aggressive Fibromatosis (Desmoid Tumour) (Fig. 78)

A locally infiltrative fibroblastic growth.

This tumour is composed of elongated fibroblasts, sometimes resembling smooth muscle cells, separated by collagen and arranged in poorly defined interlacing sweeping fascicles. The cells have bland cytologic features with uniform pale-staining nuclei and one or more small nucleoli. Mitoses are rare; there are no abnormal mitoses. Inflammatory cells are usually not present within the lesion, but perivascular lymphocytic infiltration is common at the advancing margins.

47 Angiofibroma (Juvenile Angiofibroma) (Figs. 79–81)

This tumour arises in the posterolateral nasal wall or the nasopharynx and occurs almost exclusively in young males aged 10–25 years. It is composed of vascular and fibrous elements in varying proportions. The vessels in the superficial portions of the tumour are mainly gaping capillaries which may become compressed with increasing stromal fibrosis. Thick-walled vessels without elastic membranes and with irregular, incomplete or absent muscle coats and focal intimal thickenings are usually present in the deeper portions of the tumour. The vascular elements are embedded in fibrous tissue which varies in cellularity and collagenization; stellate fibroblast-like cells are often present close to the blood vessels. The fibroblastic cells may exhibit cytologic atypia, and some of the cells may be multinucleated, but mitoses are rare. Mast cells are common and may be numerous. There may be focal thrombosis, haemorrhage and chronic inflammatory reaction. The tumour is sessile or polypoid and is histologically benign but has a tendency to recur and is locally destructive, causing pressure necrosis of adjacent soft tissue and bone and occasionally extending into paranasal sinuses, orbit and cranial fossae.

48 Myxoma (Myxofibroma) (Fig. 82)

A tumour composed of small spindle-shaped or stellate cells embedded in a myxoid matrix.

The tumour cells have small irregular hyperchromatic nuclei and fine cytoplasmic processes. The matrix is composed of abundant mucomyxoid material (Alcian blue positive, hyaluronidase labile) in a loose meshwork of reticulin and collagen fibres. The tumour is poorly vascularized. It is not well demarcated and tends to recur. The tumour usually arises in the maxilla and may involve the antrum and nasal cavity; it may very rarely arise in the soft tissues of the larynx. It should be distinguished from inflammatory sinonasal polyps (item 104), laryngeal polyps (item 105) and the myxoid variants of lipoblastic, rhabdomyoblastic and nerve sheath tumours.

49 Fibrous Histiocytoma (Fig. 83)

A benign unencapsulated tumour made up of fibroblastic and histio-cytic cells.

The fibroblastic cells are typically arranged in cartwheel or stori-form patterns. The tumour frequently contains chronic inflamma-tory cells, macrophages containing lipid or haemosiderin and Tou-ton-type giant cells. It may have a prominent vascular component. Mitoses are scarce.

50 Lipoma and Liposarcoma

The lipoma is made up of mature adipocytes; it is frequently inter-sected by bands of fibrous tissue. Lipomas undergoing myxoid changes should be distinguished from myxoma (item 48) and myx-oid liposarcoma. Liposarcomas are composed of fat cells of varying maturity and are identified by the presence of lipoblasts. They be-long to four major subgroups that differ in their histological appear-ances and biological behaviour: liposarcomas with *well-differen-tiated* (lipoma-like) or *myxoid* structure are of low-grade malignancy and those with *round cell* or *pleomorphic* structure are high-grade sarcomas.

51 Leiomyoma and Leiomyosarcoma (Figs. 84–86)

The tumour cells are usually spindle shaped with elongated blunt-ended nuclei and eosinophilic fibrillar or vacuolated cytoplasm. They are arranged in interlacing bundles with abundant intercellular reticulin. Some tumours may exhibit nuclear palisading reminiscent of neurilemmoma. In the *vascular leiomyoma* (angioleiomyoma) the bundles of smooth muscle are continuous with and appear to arise from thick-walled blood vessels which may be a major component of the neoplasm. The *epithelioid leiomyoma* is composed mainly of round or polygonal cells with clear or eosinophilic cytoplasm. The cells of smooth muscle tumours contain glycogen (PAS positive, diastase labile) and non-striated myofibrils and are usually immu-noreactive for actin, desmin and myosin. Electron microscopy re-veals thin parallel myofilaments with interspersed elliptical dense bodies, attachment plaques, rare junctions with adjacent cells and a lamina externa which may be focally discontinuous. Malignant tu-mours exhibit mitotic activity and are generally more cellular with larger hyperchromatic nuclei; necrosis is common. Leiomyomas and well-differentiated leiomyosarcomas have closely similar features and are difficult to distinguish histologically. The presence of five or more mitoses per 10 high-power fields (hpf) is usually indicative of malignancy; tumours with 1–4 mitoses per 10 hpf may be regarded as potentially malignant.

52 Rhabdomyoma (Figs. 87, 88)

A benign tumour composed of striated muscle cells.

The tumour is well circumscribed, and the component cells have eosinophilic fibrillar cytoplasm that stains positively with Masson trichrome and PTAH stains. Cross-striations may be present. The cells are immunoreactive for actin, desmin and myoglobin. By electron microscopy they usually exhibit thick and thin myofilaments and Z and I bands. Most recorded cases of this rare neoplasm have occurred in the upper neck region, tongue, pharynx and larynx. Two subtypes, fetal and adult, are recognized on the basis of their histomorphology.

52.1 Fetal Rhabdomyoma (Fig. 87)

The tumour is typically myxoid and contains varying proportions of thin elongated muscle cells with eosinophilic cytoplasm and occasional cross striations and undifferentiated mesenchymal cells with small oval or spindle shaped nuclei and scanty cytoplasm. The tumour may be predominantly *myxoid,* with the cells loosely arranged in a myxoid matrix, or predominantly *cellular,* with interlacing fascicles of closely packed immature spindle cells. The cells have a tendency to become progressively more mature from the centre to the periphery. The tumour is distinguished from embryonal rhabdomyosarcoma (item 63.1) by the absence of mitoses, necrosis or infiltrative growth. The distinction between fetal rhabdomyoma and embryonal rhabdomyosarcoma may be difficult.

52.2 Adult Rhabdomyoma (Fig. 88)

The tumour consists of large polygonal cells with abundant eosinophilic, finely granular, frequently vacuolated glycogen-containing cytoplasm in which rod-like crystalline structures may be identified. The nuclei are round and vesicular and tend to be peripherally placed; nucleoli are prominent. There are no mitoses. Cross-striations are usually present but sparse.

53 Haemangioma (Fig. 89)

A benign non-encapsulated lesion consisting of blood vessels of varing calibre.

It is not clear whether these lesions are hamartomas or neoplasms. Haemangiomas of the upper respiratory tract may be of the capillary, cavernous or venous types. The most common type is the capillary haemangioma which consists of lobules of blood-filled capillaries separated by loose connective tissue. The lesion should be distinguished from granuloma pyogenicum (item 127) which occurs more frequently in the upper respiratory tract. *Benign haemangioendothelioma*, a rare type of haemangioma occurring mainly in infancy, is characterized by closely packed sinusoidal channels and capillaries with poorly defined lumina lined by plump endothelial cells.

54 Haemangiopericytoma
and Malignant Haemangiopericytoma (Figs. 90, 91)

Tumours characterized by the proliferation of oval, polyhedral or spindle-shaped cells enmeshed by reticulin fibres and arranged about vascular channels that are lined by a single layer of endothelial cells.

The tumour contains numerous thin-walled blood vessels that are often found gaping or distorted by the surrounding tumour cells. The tumour cells, typically arranged around the blood vessels, are of uniform size with regular oval or elongated nuclei and pale cytoplasm. The cells may also be arranged in short haphazard fascicles or in sheets of closely packed cells containing compressed capillaries. Areas of poor cellularity, myxoid change and fibrosis are not uncommon. The tumour cells are entirely situated outside the capillaries which are lined by a single layer of normal-looking endothelium; this feature, well shown by reticulin staining, helps to distinguish the tumour from angiosarcoma (item 64). The distinction from other well-vascularized mesenchymal tumours is usually made by a process of exclusion. The histological distinction between benign and malignant haemangiopericytoma may be difficult. Malignant haemangiopericytomas usually exhibit cellular pleomorphism, mitotic activity or areas of necrosis. Tumours without any of these features may be regarded as potentially malignant since a few of them may infiltrate locally or metastasize. Haemangiopericytomas of the nasal cavity are generally less aggressive than those occurring elsewhere; they

exhibit a more orderly structure with minimal mitotic activity but
tend to recur after removal and may rarely metastasize.

55 Lymphangioma

A benign non-circumscribed lesion consisting of lymph vessels of varying calibre.

Lymphangiomas may coexist with haemangiomas and may be
hamartomas or developmental anomalies rather than true neoplasms. Their occurrence in the upper respiratory tract is exceptionally rare.

56 Neurilemmoma (Schwannoma) (Fig. 92)

A benign tumour of Schwann cells.

The tumour is well encapsulated and has two histologic patterns:
an Antoni type A pattern with compact bundles or interlacing fascicles of spindle cells with regimentation of nuclei in twisted rows or
palisades (Verocay bodies) and an Antoni type B pattern in which
more pleomorphic spindle cells are loosely and haphazardly
arranged within a wide-meshed microcystic fibrillar stroma. Nerve
fibres may be present in the capsule, but axons are usually not demonstrable within the tumour. Most of the tumour cells stain positively for S-100 protein and Leu-7. Electron micrographs show a network of convoluted cytoplasmic processes, dense layers of external
laminar material and poorly formed intercellular junctions; long-
spaced collagen fibres (Luse bodies) may be present. The tumour
often contains dilated or thick-walled blood vessels and may exhibit
secondary features such as perivascular hyalinization, calcification,
thrombosis, haemorrhage and cystic changes. There may be aggregates of macrophages containing lipid or haemosiderin. Some of the
tumour cells may have large pleomorphic nuclei with smudged chromatin, but mitoses are absent or scarce. Malignant transformation is
very rare.

57 Neurofibroma (Figs. 93, 94)

*A benign tumour consisting of a mixture of neurites, Schwann cells
and fibroblasts in a collagenous or mucoid matrix.*

The tumour is poorly demarcated and consists of elongated cells
arranged in streams or interlacing bundles separated by collagen.

Axons are demonstrable within the tumour by silver stains (Bodian, Bielchowski) and by electron microscopy. The Schwann cells have elongated wavy nuclei with pointed ends and are immunoreactive for S-100 protein. Cellular pleomorphism with large hyperchromatic nuclei may be present, but mitoses are rare. Some tumours contain organoid structures resembling Wagner-Meissner or Pacini corpuscles (tactile neurofibroma, pacinian neurofibroma), and some grow within and around nerve trunks giving them a thickened, tortuous or plexiform appearance (plexiform neurofibroma). Malignant transformation of neurofibroma may occur. Neurofibroma of the upper respiratory tract may occur as an isolated lesion or as part of von Recklinghausen disease (neurofibromatosis).

58 Granular Cell Tumour (Figs. 95, 96)

A tumour made up of large, round, polyhedral or spindle-shaped cells with granular eosinophilic cytoplasm.

The tumour cells have small usually centrally placed nuclei and abundant eosinophilic cytoplasm containing diastase-resistant, PAS-positive granules. They have poorly defined cell borders and are arranged in syncytial sheets, rows or small groups. Superficially located tumours are often accompanied by pseudoepitheliomatous hyperplasia of the overlying squamous epithelium. The tumour is not encapsulated and frequently extends into adjacent tissues. Most tumours are probably of Schwann cell origin; the tumour has been referred to as granular cell myoblastoma, but there is no evidence to support myoblastic origin. The tumour cells are immunoreactive for S-100 protein. Electron microscopy reveals numerous lysosomes with angulate bodies and complex granular phagosomes ("myelin figures"). The tumour is nearly always benign. The malignant granular cell tumour, an exceptionally rare neoplasm, is characterized by nuclear pleomorphism, prominent nucleoli, mitotic activity and necrosis.

59 Paraganglioma and Malignant Paraganglioma (Figs. 97–99)

Tumours of extra-adrenal paraganglia.

These tumours have an organoid pattern with aggregations of tumour cells *(Zellballen)* surrounded by a capillary network. The chief tumour cell has epithelioid features with abundant finely granular or frayed cytoplasm and a round or oval, vesicular or hyperchromatic nucleus. Spindle-shaped (sustentacular) cells may also be present. The chief cells contain argyrophil granules and react positively for chromogranin, neuron-specific enolase and various peptide hormones but not for cytokeratin or epithelial membrane antigen. Catecholamines may be demonstrated by formaldehyde fume-induced fluorescence in cryostat sections. Membrane-bound dense-core granules are consistently demonstrable by electron microscopy. Mitoses are rare. The tumour cells are typically arranged in alveolar compartments that are well demarcated with a reticulin stain; they may also be arranged in sheets and irregular infiltrates. The vascular or the parenchymal element may predominate in the histological picture. Tumours with a prominent vascular component may superficially resemble haemangioma or granulation tissue. Stromal haemosiderin deposits and chronic inflammatory reaction may be present.

The biological behaviour is seldom predictable on the basis of histology. Nuclear hyperchromatism and pleomorphism are common in both benign and malignant paraganglioma. Tumour necrosis, increased mitotic activity and vascular invasion are common in the malignant tumour. The jugulotympanic paraganglioma (glomus jugulare tumour) is locally invasive but metastasizes rarely.

60 Fibrosarcoma

A malignant tumour composed of fusiform cells producing reticulin and collagen and showing no other form of cellular differentiation.

The tumour cells have the characteristics of fibroblasts and are arranged in cellular fascicles that typically intersect to form a herringbone pattern. Intercellular reticulin fibres are prominent. The degree of differentiation is of prognostic significance. Well-differentiated tumours consist of bundles of uniform spindle cells with very few mitoses and abundant collagen; they should be distinguished from aggressive fibromatosis (item 46). Poorly differentiated tumours show increased cellularity, pleomorphism and mitotic activity with minimal collagen. The presence of a herringbone pattern as opposed to a storiform pattern and negative immunoperoxidase staining for alpha$_1$-antitrypsin and alpha$_1$-antichymotrypsin distinguish the tumour from malignant fibrous histiocytoma (item 61). The diagnosis of fibrosarcoma should be made only after other sarcomas with spindle cell structure have been excluded by examining multiple sections and the use of special stains.

61 Malignant Fibrous Histiocytoma (Fig. 100)

A malignant tumour with fibrohistiocytic features.

This is the malignant counterpart of fibrous histiocytoma (item 49) from which it is distinguished by high mitotic activity, anaplasia, infiltrative growth and frequent necrosis. The tumour is usually composed of spindle-shaped or pleomorphic cells with fibroblastic and histiocytic features. The fibroblastic cells are typically arranged in storiform or cartwheel patterns in relation to capillaries. Multinucleated tumour cells, foamy histiocytes and inflammatory cells are common. There are variations in structure and several subtypes – *pleomorphic-storiform, myxoid, angiomatoid, giant cell* and *inflammatory* – have been recognized. Some of these variants may resemble fibrosarcoma, rhabdomyosarcoma, liposarcoma or spindle cell carcinoma. Malignant fibrous histiocytoma is distinguished from these tumours by the frequent occurrence of a storiform growth pattern, positive immunoperoxidase staining for lysozyme, alpha$_1$-antitrypsin or alpha$_1$-antichymotrypsin and the absence of rhabdomyoblastic, lipoblastic or epithelial differentiation.

62 Atypical Fibroxanthoma (Atypical Fibrous Histiocytoma)

A pleomorphic fibrohistiocytic tumour occurring in the dermis.

The tumour is composed of a mixture of spindle, polyhedral and multinucleated cells arranged in poorly defined fascicles with abundant intercellular reticulin. The cells have large, hyperchromatic or bizarre nuclei and granular or foamy lipid-containing cytoplasm. Normal and abnormal mitoses are usually present. The tumour cells usually occur in a background of chronic inflammatory cells and reactive fibrosis; the adjacent skin frequently shows solar elastosis and increased vascularity. The tumour is histologically indistinguishable from pleomorphic malignant fibrous histiocytoma (item 61) but has a superficial location and is slow growing; metastases are rare. It is distinguished from desmoplastic malignant melanoma (item 92) by the absence of Fontana-positive melanin granules or a junctional melanocytic component and from spindle cell carcinoma (item 23) by the absence of squamous differentiation. The tumour cells stain positively for vimentin, alpha$_1$-antitrypsin and alpha$_1$-antichymotrypsin and are negative for keratin, HMB-45 and S-100 protein. The absence of melanosomes and desmosomes by electron microscopy is also helpful in differential diagnosis.

63 Rhabdomyosarcoma (Figs. 101–108)

A malignant mesenchymal tumour with rhabdomyoblastic differentiation.

The tumour is composed of varying proportions of undifferentiated mesenchymal cells and rhabdomyoblasts. The rhabdomyoblasts have brightly eosinophilic stringy cytoplasm and exhibit features of muscle differentiation, namely cross-striations with PTAH staining, positive reactivity for myoglobin, desmin, myosin and actin by immunoperoxidase staining and Z bands by electron microscopy. Glycogen is usually abundant and cells with vacuolated or clear cytoplasm are common. Embryonal, alveolar and pleomorphic types are recognized according to the predominant pattern.

63.1 Embryonal Rhabdomyosarcoma (Figs. 101–103)

This is the most common type of rhabdomyosarcoma in the upper respiratory tract; it occurs mainly in the first decade of life. The tumour is composed of varying proportions of small round cells resembling lymphoid cells and moderately pleomorphic, ovoid and spindle-shaped rhabdomyoblasts with hyperchromatic nuclei and varying amounts of deeply eosinophilic cytoplasm; strap-shaped, angulated and racquet-shaped cells may be present. Cross-striations may be present, but their demonstration is not essential for the diagnosis of rhabdomyosarcoma. The tumour may have areas of high cellularity especially around vessels and areas of low cellularity where the cells are arranged loosely in a myxoid stroma. There are numerous mitoses. The term *sarcoma botryoides* is applied clinically to tumours which form polypoid grape-like structures. Such tumours consist mainly of an oedematous or myxoid matrix with scanty tumour cells except for a cellular zone close to the epithelial surface. Embryonal rhabdomyosarcoma should be distinguished from other small cell tumours such as neuroblastoma, Ewing sarcoma, malignant lymphoma and small cell carcinoma.

63.2 Alveolar Rhabdomyosarcoma (Figs. 104–108)

This type tends to occur in older children and young adults. It is composed of compact, trabecular or alveolated masses of undifferentiated small cells and rhabdomyoblasts separated by fibrovascular stroma. The cells in the central part of the masses tend to be loose-lying, and those at the periphery are attached directly to the fibrous stroma without an intervening basement membrane. Multinucleated cells with peripherally placed nuclei are common. There is high mitotic activity. The tumour should be distinguished from adenocarcinoma.

63.3 Pleomorphic Rhabdomyosarcoma

This type is exceptionally rare in the upper respiratory tract. The tumour consists of large pleomorphic spindle-shaped or strap-like cells with abundant eosinophilic cytoplasm; the cells may contain myofibrils but cross-striations are uncommon. The tumour should be distinguished from malignant fibrous histiocytoma and other pleomorphocellular sarcomas.

64 Angiosarcoma (Fig. 109)

A malignant neoplasm characterized by the formation of irregular anastomosing vascular channels lined by atypical endothelial cells.

The endothelial tumour cells may be spindle-shaped or plump and epithelioid; they show varying grades of cytologic atypia and mitotic activity. The vascular channels may be narrow or dilated and are lined by one or more layers of tumour cells which may form papillae or tufts that project into the vascular lumina. Reticulin stains are helpful in outlining the vascular channels and demonstrating the intraluminal location of the tumour cells. The malignant cells may also be found in extravascular situations and may occasionally form sarcomatous sheets with minimal vascular canalization. Haemorrhage is a common feature. The factor VIII related antigen is usually demonstrable in well-differentiated tumours. Electron microscopy may reveal the Weibel-Palade bodies which are characteristic of vascular endothelium. The tumour is invasive, often multicentric and tends to metastasize widely. The presence of the characteristic anastomosing vascular channels helps to distinguish angiosarcoma from Kaposi sarcoma (item 65). The anaplastic character of the cells lining these vascular channels distinguishes the tumour from haemangiopericytoma (item 54) and other highly vascular soft tissue tumours.

65 Kaposi Sarcoma (Figs. 110, 111)

A malignant tumour composed of spindle cells forming and surrounding irregular slit-like vascular channels and spaces.

The tumour cells have endothelial or fibroblast-like features and are separated by reticulin fibres. The histological picture ranges from bland proliferations of vascular endothelium and perivascular spindle cells to frankly anaplastic tumours. The tumour often contains chronic inflammatory cells, extravasated erythrocytes, extracellular or intracellular PAS-positive hyaline globules of varying size and deposits of haemosiderin pigment. Dilated blood and lymph vessels are frequently found at the periphery. The tumour is often associated with the acquired immune deficiency syndrome (AIDS) or other immunosuppressed states. The lesions in the larynx and other parts of the upper respiratory tract are often multifocal and frequently associated with cutaneous, lymph nodal or visceral involvement. Tumours with a prominent vascular or fibroblastic component may resemble angiosarcoma (item 64) or fibrosarcoma (item 60), respectively. The clinical features and the presence of slit-like vascular spaces and extravasated red cells in Kaposi sarcoma are helpful in diagnosis.

66 Malignant Nerve Sheath Tumour (Malignant Schwannoma)

This tumour shares some of the histologic features of neurofibroma (item 57) and is distinguished from it by higher cellularity, pleomorphism, mitotic activity and infiltrative growth. The nuclei are often serpiginous, buckled or comma-shaped and may show palisading; these features and the presence of highly cellular areas alternating with poorly cellular myxoid zones help to distinguish the tumour from fibrosarcoma and other sarcomas with spindle-cell morphology. The S-100 protein is demonstrable in most cases. An attachment to a nerve trunk or association with neurofibromatosis is especially helpful in diagnosis. Very rarely there may be areas of chondroid, osseous, rhabdomyoblastic or glandular differentiation.

67 Alveolar Soft Part Sarcoma

A malignant soft tissue tumour composed of alveolated nests of large cells with vesicular nuclei, prominent nucleoli and abundant eosinophilic granular cytoplasm that often contains PAS-positive diastase-resistant crystalline material.

The tumour is usually intersected by fibrous bands and has a characteristic organoid structure with well-defined nests of cells separated by sinusoidal spaces lined by a single layer of vascular endo-

thelium. The typical alveolar pattern results from the detachment
and loss of cells in the central portions of the nests. The cells are
rounded or polyhedral and contain glycogen. The presence of rod-
shaped or needle-like PAS-positive, diastase-resistant crystalline inclusions is virtually diagnostic of the tumour. By electron microscopy these are seen as membrane-bound crystals which sometimes
have a cross-grid pattern. In some cases the tumour cells are immunoreactive for desmin and muscle-specific actin; there is growing evidence that alveolar soft part sarcoma has a myogenic phenotype, but
the precise histogenesis remains unsettled. The tumour should be
distinguished from malignant melanoma (item 92), paraganglioma
(item 59), alveolar rhabdomyosarcoma (item 63.2) and metastatic
renal carcinoma.

68 Synovial Sarcoma (Fig. 112)

*A malignant mesenchymal tumour with synovioblastic differentia-
tion.*

The tumour is usually well circumscribed but not encapsulated.
It is characteristically bimorphic with epithelial-like and fibrosarcoma-like components. The epithelioid cells are cuboidal, columnar or
polyhedral and may be arranged in compact masses devoid of reticulin or in tubular, papillary or gland-like structures containing
mucinous material that stains positively with mucicarmine, Alcian
blue or PAS. The spindle-cell fibrosarcoma-like component usually
consists of swirls of closely packed cells with a rich intercellular reticulin network. Mitoses are common. The tumour often contains
numerous mast cells and bands of dense collagen resembling osteoid; myxoid changes and foci of calcification are common. The epithelioid and spindle cell components react positively for vimentin
and often for cytokeratin and epithelial membrane antigen. They
are usually not separated by basement membranes but are clearly
distinguished by reticulin stains; their relative proportions vary considerably, and some tumours may be monophasic.

69 Ewing Sarcoma (Figs. 113, 114)

*A primitive mesenchymal tumour composed of uniform, small undif-
ferentiated cells.*

The tumour cells are closely packed and are arranged in sheets or
divided into nests or lobules by fine fibrovascular septa. The cells

have uniform round or oval nuclei with finely dispersed chromatin and small nucleoli. The cytoplasm is scanty, frequently vacuolated and usually contains glycogen. There are numerous mitoses. Widespread necrosis, myxoid changes and focal calcification are common; the persistence of viable cells around blood vessels may produce a haemangiopericytoma-like pattern. Tumours containing rosette-like structures and a large cell variant with cellular pleomorphism are also recognized. The tumour may arise in soft tissues or bone and usually occurs in children or young adults. It is rare in the upper respiratory tract, where it should be distinguished from other small cell tumours such as malignant lymphoma, embryonal rhabdomyosarcoma, haemangiopericytoma, olfactory neuroblastoma, metastatic neuroblastoma and small cell carcinoma. Histologic diagnosis is usually difficult and may be impossible in small or substantially necrotic biopsy samples. Cell imprints, immunocytologic techniques and electron microscopy are helpful and often essential in differential diagnosis.

Tumours of Bone and Cartilage

70 Chondroma (Fig. 115)

A benign tumour formed of mature cartilage.

The tumour consists of well-defined lobules of hyaline cartilage composed of evenly distributed clusters of mature cartilage cells embedded in metachromatic hyaline or mucomyxoid ground substance. In the upper respiratory tract the tumour arises most frequently from the laryngeal cartilages. It should be distinguished from elastic cartilage metaplasia (item 129) which occurs in the soft tissues of the larynx without attachment to cartilage. It may be difficult to distinguish between chondroma and well-differentiated chondrosarcoma (item 77) on histologic grounds.

71 Chondroblastoma

A benign tumour of bone characterized by the presence of chondroblasts, multinucleated giant cells, a chondroid matrix and foci of calcification.

The chondroblasts, the basic cells in this neoplasm, are rounded or polyhedral cells with round, oval or indented nuclei, distinct cell membranes and pericellular reticulin. A few typical mitoses are usually present. The giant cells are of the osteoclast type and are generally smaller than those in giant cell tumour. The chondroid matrix shows foci of calcification. The deposition of calcium in the pericellular reticulin gives a typical chicken-wire or honeycomb pattern. The occurrence of this tumour in the bones of the skull is exceptionally rare.

72 Osteoma (Fig. 116)

A slow-growing lesion consisting of mature bone with a predominantly lamellar structure.

Some of these lesions may be malformations rather than true neoplasms. Lesions in the external auditory meatus that are bilateral or multiple have been referred to as hyperostoses or exostoses. Osteomas may grow into the paranasal sinuses as bony masses of varying density; some may exhibit cortical bone at the periphery and cancellous bone with marrow spaces centrally.

73 Osteoid Osteoma

A bone lesion consisting of a small well-demarcated nidus of abnormal bone surrounded by a zone of reactive sclerotic bone.

The nidus comprises a tangled meshwork or anastomosing trabeculae of osteoid and/or woven bone, often rimmed by well-differentiated osteoblasts, in a background of highly vascular connective tissue which contains osteoclast-like giant cells and nerve fibres. The osseous elements in the central portion are usually more mature and exhibit prominent cement lines and calcification. There are no chondroid elements. The nidus is usually separated from the marginal sclerotic bone by a zone of fibrovascular tissue. Osteoid osteoma has limited growth potential and usually measures less than 1 cm in diameter.

74 Osteoblastoma

A benign tumour of bone composed of irregular trabeculae of osteoid and woven bone rimmed by osteoblasts and separated by highly vascular stroma.

The histological features are largely similar to those of osteoid osteoma (item 73). However, the tumour is invariably larger (generally more than 2 cm in diameter), tends to contain more plentiful osteoblasts and has less marginal sclerosis. The presence of prominent osteoblastic rimming of the osseous trabeculae and well-demarcated non-infiltrative margins and the absence of cartilaginous elements, anaplasia and abnormal mitoses are helpful in distinguishing the tumour from osteosarcoma (item 78). The distinction between osteoblastoma and well-differentiated osteosarcoma can be difficult and should take into account the clinical and radiological findings.

75 Ossifying Fibroma (Figs. 117, 118)

A benign but locally aggressive fibro-osseous tumour consisting of spindle-shaped fibroblastic cells arranged in a whorled pattern and containing small spicules and trabeculae of lamellar or woven bone and/or mineralized masses.

The tumour is found most frequently in the mandible or maxilla of young subjects. It is well circumcribed and may appear encapsulated. Mitoses may be present. The spicules and trabeculae of woven bone may show a lamellar structure peripherally and are frequently rimmed by osteoblasts. The term *cementifying fibroma* is applied to a variant of ossifying fibroma in which numerous small rounded heavily calcified masses (cementum or cementicles) are found in a cellular fibroblastic tumour. Ossifying fibroma, cementifying fibroma and fibrous dysplasia (item 135) often show overlapping features. The term *benign fibro-osseous lesion* is used to designate lesions that are not clearly assignable to any one of these categories.

76 Giant Cell Tumour

A tumour composed of large multinucleated osteoclast-like cells and mononuclear cells.

The mononuclear cells are plump, ovoid or spindle-shaped and have a round or oval nucleus with a single nucleolus. The giant cells have numerous (usually more than 20) nuclei which resemble those in the mononuclear cells and tend to be centrally located. They are evenly distributed throughout the tumour. Osteoid is present in some cases. Collagen formation is absent or minimal except in areas of fracture. Most tumours have bland cytologic features with mild or moderate mitotic activity and a benign clinical course. However, all giant cell tumours grow aggressively and are potentially malignant. The term *malignant giant cell tumour* has been variously applied to typical giant cell tumours that have metastasized, tumours with a predominant mononuclear cell component with frank anaplasia or high mitotic activity and tumours that have undergone sarcomatous transformation to fibrosarcoma, malignant fibrous histiocytoma or rarely osteosarcoma.

The giant cell tumour is rare in the facial bones; most of the recorded cases have occurred in the sphenoid and temporal bones. The tumour should be distinguished from giant cell reparative granuloma (item 136) which occurs more commonly in the jaw bones of young patients, the "brown tumour" of hyperparathyroidism which is associated with metabolic abnormalities and multiple bone involvement and various benign and malignant bone tumours which may contain osteoclast-like giant cells.

77 Chondrosarcoma (Figs. 119, 120)

A malignant tumour characterized by the formation of cartilage but not bone by the tumour cells.

The tumour is distinguished from chondroma (item 70) by its larger size, infiltrative growth and higher cellularity associated with pleomorphism, mitoses, nuclear irregularities and the presence of plump cells with large or double nuclei and prominent nucleoli. The cells are immunoreactive for vimentin and the S-100 protein. Chondrosarcoma frequently shows areas of calcification and enchondral ossification, but neither bone nor osteoid is formed directly by the tumour cells. The tumour is graded according to degree of differentiation and mitotic activity. Chondrosarcoma should be distinguished from chrondroblastic osteosarcoma (item 78) and chordoma (item 94).

Dedifferentiated chondrosarcoma (transformed chondrosarcoma) is a chondrosarcoma which is juxtaposed to another specific type of sarcoma, namely malignant fibrous histiocytoma, fibrosarcoma, rhabdomyosarcoma or osteosarcoma. The tumour carries a very poor prognosis.

Mesenchymal chondrosarcoma is a high-grade tumour characterized by the presence of islands of well-differentiated or immature cartilage among masses of undifferentiated round or spindle-shaped mesenchymal cells; this tumour is highly vascular and often shows a haemangiopericytoma-like pattern.

78 Osteosarcoma (Fig. 121)

A malignant tumour characterized by the direct formation of bone or osteoid tissue by the tumour cells.

The tumour cells may be spindle-shaped or pleomorphic and exhibit varying degrees of anaplasia and mitotic activity. Some well-differentiated sclerotic tumours may appear deceptively innocuous. The production of osteoid or woven bone by the tumour cells, on which histologic diagnosis depends, varies in extent and may require careful search and adequate sampling for identification. Cartilage formation is common and may be extensive in tumours arising in the jaw bones. This chondroblastic variant of osteosarcoma is distinguished from chondrosarcoma (item 77) by the direct formation of osteoid or woven bone by the tumour cells. Undifferentiated tumours without demonstrable bone or osteoid formation may resemble fibrosarcoma or malignant fibrous histiocytoma. Osteosarcoma produces abundant alkaline phosphatase; the demonstration of this enzyme in cell imprints or cryostat sections is helpful in diagnosis.

79 Ewing Sarcoma

See item 69.

Malignant Lymphomas

80 Malignant Lymphomas (ML) (Figs. 122–128)

The upper respiratory tract is a common site for the occurrence of extranodal lymphomas. The tumours appear as nodular polypoid masses or as diffuse infiltrates that thicken the mucosa; necrosis and ulceration are common. Lymphomas of the upper respiratory tract occur either as a primary disease or as a secondary involvement in cases of nodal lymphoma.

The overwhelming majority of upper respiratory tract lymphomas are non-Hodgkin lymphomas (NHL). They may be classified according to the NCI Working Formulation (Table 1) or the Kiel classification (Table 2) and categorized as tumours of B- or T-cell lineage by immunotyping.

Table 1. Non-Hodgkin lymphomas: NCI Working Formulation

Low grade	*High grade*

A. Malignant lymphoma
   Small lymphocytic
      Consistent with CLL
      Plasmacytoid
B. Malignant lymphoma, follicular
   Predominantly small cleaved cell
      Diffuse areas
      Sclerosis
C. Malignant lymphoma, follicular
   Mixed, small cleaved and large cell
      Diffuse areas
      Sclerosis
	H. Malignant lymphoma
	   Large cell, immunoblastic
	      Plasmacytoid
	      Clear cell
	      Polymorphous
	      Epithelioid cell component
	I. Malignant lymphoma
	   Lymphoblastic
	      Convoluted cell
	      Non-convoluted cell
	J. Malignant lymphoma
	   Small non-cleaved cell
	      Burkitt's
	      Follicular areas

Intermediate grade
 	
D. Malignant lymphoma, follicular
   Predominantly large cell
      Diffuse areas
      Sclerosis
E. Malignant lymphoma, diffuse
   Small cleaved cell
      Sclerosis
F. Malignant lymphoma, diffuse
   Mixed, small and large cell
      Sclerosis
      Epithelioid cell component
G. Malignant lymphoma, diffuse
   Large cell
      Cleaved cell
      Non-cleaved cell
      Sclerosis
	Miscellaneous
	   Composite
	   Mycosis fungoides
	   Histiocytic
	   Extramedullary plasmacytoma
	   Unclassifiable
	   Other

From Cancer 49: 2112–2135, 1982

Sinonasal T-cell lymphomas are generally associated with more marked tissue destruction than are B-cell tumours. Cases with a mixed cellular composition and an angiocentric or angioinvasive growth pattern have been termed midline malignant reticulosis (item 83).

Some upper respiratory tract lymphomas arise from mucosa-associated lymphoid tissue (MALT). These low-grade B-cell lymphomas are composed of centrocyte-like marginal zone cells and may show follicular preservation; the tumour cells tend to invade glandular and surface epithelium forming characteristic lymphoepithelial lesions.

Table 2. Non-Hodgkin lymphomas – Updated Kiel classification[1]

B-cell	T-cell
Low-grade malignant lymphomas	

Lymphocytic
  Chronic lymphocytic leukaemia
  Prolymphocytic leukaemia
  Hairy-cell leukaemia
	Lymphocytic
	  Chronic lymphocytic leukaemia
	  Prolymphocytic leukaemia

	Small cell, cerebriform Mycosis fungoides, Sezary's syndrome
Lymphoplasmacytic/-cytoid (immunocytoma)	Lymphoepithelioid (Lennert's lymphoma)
Plasmacytic	Angioimmunoblastic (AILD, LgX)

Centroblastic-centrocytic
  follicular ± diffuse
  diffuse
	T-zone lymphoma

Centrocytic	Pleomorphic, small cell (HTLV-I ±)
Monocytoid	
High-grade malignant lymphomas	
Centroblastic	Pleomorphic, medium-sized and large cell (HTLV-I ±)
Immunoblastic	Immunoblastic (HTLV-I ±)
Large cell, anaplastic (Ki-1 +)	Large cell, anaplastic (Ki-1 +)
Burkitt lymphoma	
Lymphoblastic	Lymphoblastic
Rare types	*Rare types*

[1] Lennert K, Feller AC. Histopathology of Non-Hodgkin-Lymphomas (according to the updated Kiel-classification). Springer-Verlag, Berlin Heidelberg. Second edition, 1991.

81 Non-Hodgkin Lymphoma (Conventional Types)
(Figs. 122–124)

The types of lymphoma arising in Waldeyer ring are mainly mixed small and large cell (centroblastic-centrocytic), large cell cleaved and non-cleaved (centroblastic), small cell lymphocytic with plasmacytoid differentiation and small cell lymphocytic. The types of lymphoma arising elsewhere in the upper respiratory tract are mainly large cell cleaved and non-cleaved (centroblastic), large cell immunoblastic, small cell lymphocytic with plasmacytoid differentiation, mixed small and large cell (centroblastic-centrocytic) and lymphoblastic. Secondary involvement of the upper respiratory tract occurs more frequently with NHL of the lymphoblastic, immunoblastic and follicle centre cell types. The jaw bones are frequently involved in Burkitt lymphoma in countries where the disease is endemic. The salient characteristics of these types are given below.

Malignant Lymphoma, Small Cell Lymphocytic (ML Lymphocytic). A diffuse lymphoma, usually of B-cell type, in which more than 80% of cells are small lymphocytes resembling those in chronic lymphocytic leukaemia. A vaguely nodular pattern may be mimicked by "proliferation centres" containing slightly enlarged cells with nucleoli and mitoses.

Malignant Lymphoma, Small Cell Lymphocytic with Plasmacytoid Differentiation (ML Lymphoplasmacytoid). A diffuse lymphoma of B-cell type composed of small lymphocytes and plasmacytoid lymphocytes. The latter have the nuclear morphology of lymphocytes, amphophilic or basophilic cytoplasm and occasional intracytoplasmic or intranuclear PAS-positive immunoglobulin inclusions.

Malignant Lymphoma, Follicular, Mixed Small Cleaved and Large Cell (ML Centroblastic-Centrocytic, Follicular ± Diffuse). These tumours have a follicular or nodular pattern with areas of diffuse growth and are composed of a mixture of small cleaved cells and large cleaved or non-cleaved cells. The tumours are usually of B-cell type and characteristically have variable amounts of pale cytoplasm and hypochromatic nuclei with nucleoli at the nuclear membranes.

Malignant Lymphoma, Mixed Small and Large Cell, Diffuse (ML Centroblastic-Centrocytic, Diffuse). An immunologically heterogenous group of tumours of mixed cellular composition with small lymphocytes, cleaved cells and large blasts. There may be a plasmacytoid component, and the blasts may include multinucleated immunoblasts.

Malignant Lymphoma, Large Cell Cleaved and Non-cleaved, Diffuse (ML Centroblastic-Centrocytic, Diffuse and ML Centroblastic). These B-cell tumours are related to the follicle cell lymphomas but are composed primarily of large pale-staining cells with a predominantly diffuse growth pattern. There may be foci of sclerosis.

Malignant Lymphoma, Large Cell Immunoblastic (ML Immunoblastic). A diffuse lymphoma with predominance of large cells of B-

or T-cell type with round or oval vesicular nuclei, prominent single nucleoli and amphophilic or basophilic cytoplasm. Plasmacytoid, clear cell and pleomorphic variants may be recognized. The pleomorphic variant is composed of small lymphoid cells with twisted nuclei and large cells with clear cytoplasm and multiple or lobated nuclei resembling the Reed-Sternberg cells of Hodgkin disease; aggregates of plasma cells and epithelioid cells may be present.

Malignant Lymphoma, Lymphoblastic, Convoluted or Non-convoluted (ML Lymphoblastic). A diffuse lymphoma of medium-sized lymphoid cells of B-, T- or U-cell type with deeply staining nuclei with finely dispersed granular chromatin, small nucleoli and scanty grey or basophilic cytoplasm. The nuclei may be round (non-convoluted) or folded (convoluted). There may or may not be a "starry sky" appearance due to the presence of macrophages containing nuclear debris.

Malignant Lymphoma, Small Non-cleaved Cell, Burkitt (Burkitt Lymphoma). A B-cell lymphoma composed of dense sheets of intermediate-sized lymphoblasts with a prominent "starry sky" pattern due to the presence of macrophages containing nuclear debris. The lymphoblasts have round nuclei with coarsely reticulated chromatin and multiple nucleoli. Their narrow cytoplasmic rims are basophilic and contain lipid droplets.

Small cell lymphomas with minimal cytologic atypia may resemble lymphoid hyperplasia (item 138) and inflammatory infiltrates containing reactive immunoblasts; they may be distinguished by their monomorphism, infiltrative growth with invasion of glandular or crypt epithelium and monoclonality as shown by immunotyping. Small cell lymphomas with obvious cytologic atypia may resemble small cell carcinoma (item 43), embryonal rhabdomyosarcoma (item 63.1), Ewing sarcoma (item 69) or olfactory neuroblastoma (item 93); immunostaining for the leucocyte common antigen, keratin, desmin, chromogranin and neuron-specific enolase are helpful in differential diagnosis. Large cell lymphomas may resemble nasopharyngeal undifferentiated carcinoma (item 27.2.2) or amelanotic melanoma (item 92); they may be distinguished by their respective immunoreactivities for the leucocyte common antigen, keratin and S-100 protein or HMB-45.

82 Extramedullary Plasmacytoma
(Extramedullary Plasmacytic Lymphoma) (Fig. 125)

An extramedullary lymphoma formed exclusively of plasma cells in varying degrees of differentiation.

The upper respiratory tract is the most frequent site of extramedullary plasmacytoma; the tumour occurs most commonly in the nasal cavity and sinuses. While presenting in the upper respiratory tract the tumour may later prove to be part of a systemic disease. The tumour cells vary from normal-looking plasma cells to less mature cells which are more pleomorphic and have larger and more centrally placed nuclei. Binuclear forms may be present. The cells stain positively with the methyl green-pyronine stain. By electron microscopy they show plentiful rough endoplasmic reticulum and a prominent Golgi apparatus.

The tumour cells are arranged in sheets that are intersected and often compartmentalized by delicate vascular stroma. Deposits of amyloid may be present. The condition is distinguished from plasma cell granuloma (item 139) by the absence of inflammatory cells except near ulcerated surfaces, the immaturity of the cells and especially by their monoclonality as shown by the presence of only one of the classes of light chains by immunostaining. Extramedullary plasmacytoma is a low-grade lymphoma with relatively favourable prognosis.

83 Midline Malignant Reticulosis (Polymorphic Reticulosis, Lymphomatoid Granulomatosis) (Figs. 126–128)

A necrotizing, angiocentric or angioinvasive lymphoma that occurs as a slowly progressing destructive disease in the upper respiratory tract.

The lesion is characterized by a mixed cellular infiltrate comprising small and large neoplastic lymphoid cells, some resembling activated lymphocytes or blasts and many with tortuous nuclei and clear cytoplasm, admixed with granulocytes, macrophages and plasma cells. Mitoses are common. The tumour cells are angiocentric or angioinvasive, and there may be thrombosis of small vessels. True vasculitis with fibrinoid necrosis and giant cell granulomas are generally absent. There is widespread coagulative necrosis. The lesion occurs most frequently in the sinonasal tract, nasopharynx and palate and less frequently in the larynx. It is ulcerative and locally destructive and may involve contiguous structures with erosion of bone and facial ulceration in some cases. The clinical course is not unlike conventional extranodal lymphoma, and systemic involvement is common in untreated cases. The histological features have a close resemblance to pulmonary lymphomatoid granulomatosis.

The long-standing controversy regarding the nature of midline malignant (polymorphic) reticulosis has been compounded by the use of diverse terminology without standardized diagnostic criteria. Because the necrotizing character of the lesion and its mixed cellular composition did not fit well with any of the conventional types of lymphoma the disease has been previously categorized as a non-neoplastic or pre-lymphomatous lymphoproliferative disorder. With more uniform diagnostic criteria and the use of lymphoid cell markers it is now widely recognized that midline malignant reticulosis is a type of malignant lymphoma and that the overwhelming majority is of peripheral T-cell origin.

Note: The term *lethal midline granuloma* has been applied clinically to a heterogenous group of midfacial destructive diseases involving the upper respiratory tract. Causes of this syndrome include infective granulomas (item 109), Wegener granulomatosis (item 110) midline malignant reticulosis (polymorphic reticulosis) (item 83), malignant histiocytosis (item 84) and the conventional types of non-Hodgkin lymphoma (item 81). In distinguishing between these lesions it is essential to have adequate biopsy specimens including viable tissue adjoining the necrotic areas. The term *idiopathic midline destructive disease* has been applied clinically to cases without systemic involvement in which clinical, microbiologic and histologic examinations have not established any of the causes of the lethal midline granuloma syndrome. Histologic examination in such cases reveals only non-specific inflammatory, necrotic and reactive changes, i. e. without infective agents, primary vasculitis or cytologic atypia.

84 Histiocytic Lymphomas

True histiocytic lymphoma, composed of cells derived from the monocyte-macrophage system, may rarely occur in the upper respiratory tract. The tumour cells have oval or lobated nuclei, multiple small nucleoli and abundant cytoplasm with well-defined cell margins. They may exhibit phagocytic activity and react positively for lysozyme, alpha$_1$-antitrypsin and alpha$_1$-antichymotrypsin.

Malignant histiocytosis (histiocytic medullary reticulosis) is a systemic disease characterized by infiltration by pleomorphic histiocytes with bizarre nuclei, prominent nucleoli and abnormal mitoses. Multinucleated cells may be present. The tumour cells exhibit erythrophagocytosis and react positively for lysozyme, alpha$_1$-antitrypsin and alpha₁-antichymotrypsin. Lesions in the upper respiratory tract may be associated with the so-called lethal midline granuloma syndrome (see note under item 83).

85 Hodgkin Disease

A form of lymphoma characterized by the presence of the Reed-Sternberg cell and its variants.

The classical Reed-Sternberg cell is a large cell with abundant pale amphophilic cytoplasm and lobated or multiple nuclei with a very large eosinophilic nucleolus surrounded by a halo in each lobe or nucleus. The disease is subdivided into four histological types characterized by *lymphocyte predominance, nodular sclerosis, mixed cellularity* and *lymphocyte depletion,* respectively. Hodgkin disease occurs infrequently in Waldeyer ring and is exceptionally rare in other parts of the upper respiratory tract.

Miscellaneous Tumours

86 Melanocytic Naevus (Fig. 129)

This lesion consists of nests, loose aggregates or fascicles of naevus cells that may be situated in the dermis (dermal naevus), lower epidermis at the dermo-epidermal interface (junctional naevus) or both locations (compound naevus). The cells may be epithelioid, rounded, cuboidal or spindle-shaped and generally have uniform ovoid nuclei without prominent nucleoli; multinucleated cells may be present. There may be areas of neuroid differentiation. The naevus cells usually contain melanin pigment (Fontana positive) and are immunoreactive for HMB-45 and S-100 protein.

87 Meningioma (Figs. 130, 131)

Extracranial meningiomas may be predominantly meningothelial (syncytical), fibroblastic, transitional or psammomatous; their histological features are similar to those of intracranial meningioma. The type occurring most frequently in the upper respiratory tract and ear is the meningothelial, which is composed of plump spindle-shaped cells often arranged in concentric onion-skin-like whorls with or without formation of psammoma bodies. The cells have regular round or oval frequently folded nuclei with finely dispersed chromatin and pale cytoplasm with poorly defined cell margins. Nests and sheets of polyhedral cells may also be present. The tumour cells are usually immunoreactive for vimentin and epithelial membrane antigen and occasionally for cytokeratin and S-100 protein. By electron microscopy they have numerous branching interdigitating cytoplasmic processes joined by desmosomes. The tumour may represent a local extension from an intracranial tumour or a primary arising from ectopic meningeal tissue in the sinonasal tract, nasopharynx, temporal bone or middle ear.

88 Ameloblastoma (Fig. 132)

A variety of odontogenic tumours may extend into the sinonasal tract; they may also occur as primary tumours in the maxillary antrum. Ameloblastoma, the most common of these tumours, is a locally invasive tumour composed of follicular or plexiform cell masses separated by fibrous stroma. The cell masses have central zones of loosely packed cells resembling a stellate reticulum surrounded by a single row of columnar cells with nuclei typically polarized away from the basement membrane. Some tumours exhibit basaloid, squamous or granular cell features. The stroma bordering the cell masses is often hyalinized. Cystic changes are common within the cell masses and in the connective tissue stroma.

89 Melanotic Neuroectodermal Tumour (Melanotic Progonoma) (Figs. 133, 134)

This rare tumour, probably of neural crest derivation, occurs most commonly in the maxilla of young infants. The tumour is bimorphic with varying proportions of small hyperchromatic neuroblast-like cells containing dense-core granules and larger cuboidal cells which have paler nuclei and often contain abundant melanin granules. The neuroblast-like cells are often admixed with neurofibrillary material and are sometimes found within alveolar spaces lined by the melanin-containing cells. The tumour cells are arranged in nests, cords and alveolar spaces separated by abundant fibrous stroma. They are immunopositive for neuron-specific enolase and S-100 protein. The tumour is non-encapsulated, rapidly growing and locally aggressive; it usually has a benign clinical course but may recur after removal and very rarely metastasizes.

90 Craniopharyngioma (Fig. 135)

A tumour of vestigial remnants of the craniopharyngeal duct (Rathke pouch).

The neoplasm arises within or above the sella and may rarely extend downwards to involve the nasopharynx. It consists of irregular masses and thick branching ribbons of stratified epithelium separated by loose connective tissue stroma. The cells in the central portions of the epithelial masses appear stellate and the peripheral columnar or basal cells bordering the stroma show palisading reminiscent of ameloblastoma. Intercellular oedema is usually present and may progress to cyst formation; cysts may also develop from stromal degeneration. Squamous epithelium, masses of keratin, cholesterol clefts, haemosiderin granules and calcification are common features. Craniopharyngiomas may be predominantly cystic or solid.

91 Mature Teratomas (Teratoid Tumours) (Fig. 136)

Tumours or tumour-like malformations composed of a variety of mature tissues that are foreign to their sites of occurrence and typically derived from more than one germ layer.

Benign teratoid tumours of the upper respiratory tract are for the most part developmental malformations rather than true neoplasms; they are rare and are most commonly encountered in infancy.

The *dermoid cyst* is composed of one or more cysts lined by mature keratinizing stratified squamous epithelium with skin appendages.

The *hairy polyp* is a solid polypoid lesion covered by skin with hairs and sebaceous glands. It consists mainly of fibroadipose tissue; foci of muscle, bone or cartilage are occasionally present. The lesion is found attached to the palate or nasopharynx.

The *typical teratoma* consists of tissues derived from at least two of the three germinal layers. The term *epignathus* has been applied to a bizarre mass of tissue resembling a parasitic fetus with poorly formed organs or limbs. This rare congenital lesion is usually found attached to the sphenoid, nasopharynx or palate.

92 Malignant Melanoma (Fig. 137)

Malignant melanomas occurring in the upper respiratory tract exhibit the same range of structure found in those arising in the skin but have a poorer prognosis. They may be primary or metastatic. Primary tumours may be recognized by the presence of junctional activity and/or an intraepithelial component in the adjacent mucosa; these features may be lost in the more advanced stages of the disease. The tumour cells may be spindle-shaped, polyhedral or pleomorphic and usually have finely granular cytoplasm and prominent eosinophilic nucleoli. The cells grow in loosely cohesive sheets, fascicles or pseudo-alveolar patterns. A rare balloon cell variant with clear cytoplasm may mimic clear cell carcinoma. Most tumours have cells containing melanin pigment that may be identified by silver stains (Fontana). The diagnosis of tumours in which melanin is not demonstrable by light microscopy (amelanotic melanoma) is assisted by immunoperoxidase staining by which the cells are positive for HMB-45 and S-100 protein or by electron microscopy which reveals the presence of premelanosomes and/or melanosomes.

93 Olfactory Neuroblastoma (Figs. 138–144)

A malignant neoplasm composed of neuroblasts of olfactory membrane origin.

The tumour arises exclusively in the upper part of the nasal cavity in areas corresponding with the distribution of the olfactory epithelium, i.e. the roof of nose, cribriform plate, superior nasal turbinate and upper part of the nasal septum. It has a bimodal age distribution with peaks in the 2nd and 6th decades.

Characteristically, the tumour has a lobular pattern with well-defined groups of neuroblasts and neurofibrils separated by highly vascular fibrous stroma. Foci of necrosis and dystrophic calcification may be present. The neuroblasts are seen as small uniform cells with round or oval dark nuclei with evenly distributed chromatin with or without discernible nucleoli. They have poorly defined cytoplasm and are usually separated by fibrillar material in which axons are demonstrable by silver stains (Bodian, Bielchowski). Some of the cells may contain argyrophil granules (Grimelius positive), and a few may contain Fontana-positive pigment. Most of the tumour cells are immunoreactive for neuron-specific enolase and some, especially at the periphery of the tumour masses, are also positive for S-100 protein. Some tumours contain cells that are positive for chromogranin, neurofilaments and cytokeratin. In rare instances catecholamines may be demonstrated by formaldehyde fume-induced fluorescence. Neuritic processes, neurotubules and membrane-bound dense-core granules are demonstrable by electron microscopy; some of the cells are joined with tight junctions and desmosomes.

The tumour cells may be arranged around capillaries (perivascular rosettes) or around spaces containing neurofibrillary material (Homer Wright rosettes). Some tumours contain true olfactory (Flexner-type) rosettes with well-defined lumina lined by columnar cells resembling olfactory epithelium; these cells generally have basally situated nuclei and merge with the adjacent neuroblasts without any intervening basal lamina. In some cases the tumour cells are closely associated with the epithelial components of the nasal mucosa. There is little agreement on whether these variations in structure represent differences in histogenesis or biological behaviour.

Well-differentiated olfactory neuroblastoma (grade 1), associated with good prognosis, is composed of uniform cells with bland nuclei, little or no mitotic activity and abundant neurofibrils. Anaplastic neuroblastoma (grade 4), associated with aggressive growth and very poor prognosis, is a highly cellular neoplasm with anisonucleosis, high mitotic activity and little or no evidence of neurofibrils or rosette formation. Tumours with intermediate degrees of differentiation, cellularity and mitotic activity (grades 2 and 3) comprise the majority. Most neuroblastomas with epithelial components are grade 2 neoplasms, and most of those with Flexner-type rosettes belong to grade 3.

Olfactory neuroblastoma should be distinguished from other small cell tumours occurring in this region such as small cell carcinoma (item 43), rhabdomyosarcoma (item 63), Ewing sarcoma (item 69), malignant lymphomas (item 80) and malignant melanoma (item 92).

In some olfactory neuroblastomas the tumour cells are closely attached to and appear to arise from the basal cells and seromucinous glands of the nasal mucosa. These epithelial components appear to participate in the neoplastic process but are not found in metastases. Neurofibrils are generally absent or scarce in this type of tumour which tends to occur more frequently in the older age groups. It has been suggested that such tumours may represent a type of neuroendocrine carcinoma.

94 Chordoma (Figs. 145, 146)

A tumour of notochordal origin composed of lobular masses of pleo-morphic vacuolated cells occurring in a mucoid or myxoid matrix.

This rare neoplasm occurs mainly in relation to the axial skeleton. Tumours arising in the spheno-occipital region may involve the nasopharynx and, less frequently, the nasal cavity and sinuses. The most characteristic type of tumour cell is a voluminous polyhedral cell with well-defined cell margins and markedly vacuolated bubbly cytoplasm (physaliphorous cell); the vacuoles may be empty or contain glycogen or mucoid material. Fusiform or stellate cells and non-vacuolated cells with eosinophilic cytoplasm also occur. The tumour cells are sometimes pleomorphic and may exhibit nuclear atypia, but mitoses are scarce. The tumour is frequently intersected by bands of fibrous tissue and has a characteristic lobular structure. Within individual lobules the cells are arranged in sheets, irregular clusters or trabeculae separated by mucoid material which occasionally forms lakes. There may be foci of calcification and haemorrhage. The tumour is often partially encapsulated but is infiltrative and recurs after removal. Metastases are rare. Some spheno-occipital chordomas exhibit focal chondroid differentiation; this subgroup, termed chondroid chordoma, has been associated with longer survivals. Immunoperoxidase stains are helpful in distinguishing the tumour from chondrosarcoma, liposarcoma and mucinous adenocarcinoma. Chordomas stain positively for cytokeratin, epithelial membrane antigen, vimentin and S-100 protein whereas chondrosarcomas and liposarcomas are negative for cytokeratin and epithelial membrane antigen and mucinous adenocarcinomas are negative for vimentin and S-100 protein. The presence of desmosomes and cytoplasmic tonofilaments in chordomas is also helpful in distinguishing the tumour from chondrosarcoma.

95 Malignant Germ Cell Tumours (Figs. 147–150)

Various germ cell tumours with histologic features similar to those occurring in the gonads may rarely arise in the upper respiratory tract and ear, usually in infancy and early childhood. The *immature teratoma* contains immature (embryonic) tissues, mainly of neural origin, in addition to mature tissues derived from the three embryonic germ layers; mitoses are present in the immature elements. The *teratoma with malignant transformation* is a teratoma containing a specific type of malignant tumour, e. g. squamous cell carcinoma, adenocarcinoma or sarcoma. The *yolk sac tumour* (endodermal sinus tumour) is composed of a loose meshwork of flattened or plump cuboidal primitive cells arranged in microcystic, reticular or papillary patterns and forming characteristic perivascular Schiller-Duval bodies. The cells have atypical nuclei and clear or vacuolated glycogen-containing cytoplasm. Intracellular and extracellular eosinophilic PAS-positive, diastase-resistant hyaline globules are present. Necrosis is common. There are numerous mitoses. By immunostaining the cells are positive for cytokeratin, alpha$_1$-antitrypsin and alpha-fetoprotein.

The term *teratocarcinosarcoma* has been applied to tumours occurring in adults characterized by the presence of benign and malignant epithelial, mesenchymal and neural elements including immature tissues with blastomatous features. It is questionable whether this tumour is of germ cell origin; the histogenesis is not settled. The tumour may contain microcysts lined by squamous and/or columnar epithelium, glandular structures, a spectrum of mesenchymal tissues of varying maturity with foci of myxoid appearance and neural tissues forming rosettes and neuroblastoma-like masses. Tubular epithelium-lined organoid structures surrounded by smooth muscle are common. The tumour occurs mainly in the ethmoid and other paranasal sinuses, grows aggressively and has poor prognosis.

Secondary Tumours

96 Secondary Tumours

These may be direct extensions of cancers arising in other sites in the head and neck or metastases from cancers of distant organs – most commonly from malignant melanoma and carcinomas of the kidney, breast and lung and less frequently from carcinomas of the gastrointestinal and genito-urinary tracts.

Unclassified Tumours

97 Unclassified Tumours

These are benign and malignant tumours that cannot be placed in any of the categories described above.

Tumour-like Lesions

98 Cysts (Fig. 151)

Developmental cysts of branchial cleft origin occur in the lateral wall of the nasopharynx or external ear and those derived from the embryonal pharyngeal bursa or median pharyngeal recess occur in the midline of the nasopharynx (Thornwaldt bursa). These cysts are lined by squamous and/or columnar ciliated epithelium. Cysts of second branchial cleft origin characteristically contain abundant lymphoid tissue, including germinal centres, in their walls; those of first branchial cleft origin which generally occur about the ear, angle of mandible and parotid region are usually devoid of lymphoid tissue.

Epidermoid cysts are lined by keratinizing stratified squamous epithelium and are often filled with keratin. They are distinguished from dermoid cysts (item 91) by the absence of dermal adnexal elements. Epidermoid cysts may result from an error in development or from trauma (implantation cyst).

Retention cysts are brought about by obstruction of ducts of seromucinous glands. They are usually lined by flattened or cuboidal epithelium and may contain mucinous or purulent material. Rupture of the cysts leads to extravasation of their mucinous contents and the formation of pseudocysts (mucoceles, mucus extravasation cysts) which contain mucin and muciphages and are limited by granulation tissue. Retention cysts in the larynx are lined by cuboidal or columnar epithelium which may show squamous or oncocytic metaplasia.

Saccular cysts are cystic dilatations of the laryngeal saccule which contain mucus and do not communicate with the laryngeal lumen; they differ from laryngoceles which are air-filled dilatations of the saccule that communicate with the laryngeal lumen. Saccular cysts may be congenital or acquired. They are lined by respiratory epithelium which may contain a variable number of goblet cells; foci of stratified squamous epithelium may be present.

99 Mucocele of the Paranasal Sinuses

This is a retention phenomenon of the paranasal sinuses which results in a cystic cavity lined by sinus epithelium. The contents are generally mucinous but may be hemorrhagic or purulent. Mucoceles may cause pressure destruction of the adjacent bony walls.

Inspissated mucus may form rubbery greyish brown masses in the sinonasal tract. Histologically the mass consists of mucoid material with entrapped inflammatory cells and desquamated epithelium in varying stages of disintegration. This lesion is a complication of chronic sinusitis; some cases are associated with aspergillosis (item 109).

100 Accessory Tragus (Accessory Auricle)

A sessile or pedunculated polypoid lesion located in front of the external ear.

Accessory tragi are covered by skin and usually contain cartilage, thereby simulating the structure of the external ear. The lesion represents a congenital developmental anomaly; it may be unilateral or bilateral and single or multiple.

101 Hamartoma

A developmental anomaly characterized by the formation of a tumour-like mass composed of mature tissue elements that are normally present in the location where it is found but occurring in abnormal proportions or arrangement.

A hamartoma may resemble a benign neoplasm, e. g. haemangioma, lipoma or chondroma, when only one tissue is identified.

102 Heterotopia (Choristoma)

A developmental anomaly characterized by the presence of mature tissue elements that are not normally present in the location where it is found.

102.1 Heterotopic Thyroid Tissue

Mature thyroid follicles may occur in ectopic sites such as the laryngotracheal mucosa. This lesion, a developmental abnormality, is usually a chance finding in laryngectomy specimens or at necropsy but may rarely form tumour-like masses associated with obstructive symptoms. In cases where the thyroid follicles contain little or no colloid the diagnosis may be confirmed by immunoperoxidase staining for thyroglobulin. The possibility of spread form a well-differentiated follicular carcinoma or the follicular variant of papillary carcinoma of the thyroid should be excluded clinically.

102.2 Heterotopic Salivary Gland

This lesion occurs as a mass of seromucinous glands comprising secretory and ductal elements resembling salivary gland tissue.

102.3 Heterotopic Brain Tissue
(Glial Heterotopia, "Nasal Glioma") (Figs. 152, 153)

This lesion usually occurs about the base of the nose or in the upper part of the nasal cavity. It is usually composed of astrocytes, glial fibres and fibrous connective tissue. PTAH staining for glial fibres and immunostaining for glial fibrillary acidic protein are helpful in diagnosis. Many of the glial cells have large nuclei resembling nerve cells, and some may be multinucleated. A few nerve cells or ependymal elements may rarely be identified. There are no mitoses. The lesion occurs in young children and is usually congenital. It is a developmental abnormality which may be a variant of meningo-encephalocele (item 103); the commonly used synonym "nasal glioma" is therefore a misnomer.

102.4 Heterotopic Pituitary Tissue

This lesion is an incidental finding in the posterosuperior wall of the nasopharynx or the sphenoid bone. It is composed of cells with histologic and immunocytologic features similar to those of the anterior lobe of pituitary gland. The lesion may resemble ectopic pituitary adenoma (item 11) histologically but does not produce a clinically apparent mass or hormonal disorder.

103 Meningocele and Meningo-encephalocele

Extracranial extrusions or herniations of the meninges and/or brain tissue.

In the upper respiratory tract these lesions may occur in the nasal cavity, nasofrontal region and nasopharynx. A demonstrable connection with the central nervous system and/or the presence of a fluid-filled sac distinguishes these lesions from heterotopic brain tissue (item 102.3).

104 Inflammatory Sinonasal Polyps (Figs. 154, 155)

Polypoid projections of sinonasal mucosa with variable inflammatory changes.

Nasal polyps arise most frequently in the ethmoidal region and the upper part of the nasal cavity. Those arising in the maxillary antrum may extend into the middle meatus and project anteriorly (antronasal polyps) or posteriorly (antrochoanal polyps).

The polyps consist largely of myxoid oedematous tissue in which pseudocysts containing eosinophilic proteinaceous fluid and infiltrates of inflammatory cells may be identified. The polyps are covered by respiratory epithelium with variable ulceration, goblet cell hyperplasia, squamous metaplasia and thickening of the basement membranes. Seromucous glands and mucin-containing cysts may also occur. Epithelial dysplasia is present in a few cases. Fibrosis is common and metaplastic bone formation occurs rarely in longstanding lesions. Granulomas may be present in polyps treated with intranasal injection or application of steroids or other oily medications. Atypical fibroblasts or histiocytes with abundant cytoplasm, poorly defined cell borders and large hyperchromatic occasionally pleomorphic or multilobated nuclei and prominent nucleoli are present in a small proportion of cases; these cells occur individually rather than in cohesive aggregates and are more frequently found close to blood vessels or near the epithelial surface. Such stromal atypia is a reactive phenomenon which should not be confused with sarcoma. Mitoses are scarce.

Most nasal polyps are of allergic origin; some are of infective, chemical or metabolic aetiology. Nasal polyps associated with mucoviscidosis contain cystic glands filled with inspissated mucoid material. Allergic polyps usually exhibit heavy infiltration by eosinophils, marked thickening of the basement membranes and goblet cell hyperplasia. The histological appearances of nasal polyps do not always correlate well with their aetiology.

105 Vocal Cord Nodule and Polyp (Figs. 156–158)

Nodular or polypoid lesions of the vocal cord representing stromal reactions to injury.

The terms vocal cord nodule and vocal cord polyp are generally used synonymously on account of their closely similar and overlapping histologic features. These lesions are sometimes distinguished on the basis of their clinical characteristics.

Vocal cord nodules are sessile fusiform swellings that are typically bilateral and found near the junction of the anterior and middle third of the vocal cords. They consist of avascular fibrous tissue covered by hyperplastic squamous epithelium.

Vocal cord polyps are typically unilateral spherical lesions that may be attached to any part of the vocal cord. They may be predominantly oedematous (myxoid), fibrous, vascular or hyaline; most polyps exhibit mixed appearances. Early lesions usually show oedema and fibroblastic proliferation. Well-developed lesions contain numerous thin- and thick-walled blood vessels which may be dilated and filled with hyalinized thrombi. Haemorrhage and aggregates of hemosiderin pigment are common. There is exudation of fibrin and deposition of eosinophilic hyaline material resembling amyloid around blood vessels and in the stroma. Some lesions have a predominantly collagenous or myxoid structure. Vocal cord polyps are covered by stratified squamous epithelium that may be atrophic, hyperplastic, keratotic or parakeratotic. Epithelial dysplasia is uncommon.

106 Inflammatory Otic (Aural) Polyp (Figs. 159, 160)

A polypoid lesion in the auditory meatus or middle ear consisting of inflammatory granulation tissue covered by ciliated columnar or squamous epithelium.

This lesion frequently originates in the middle ear as a complication of otitis media and projects into the auditory meatus through a perforated tympanic membrane. The surface epithelium is usually ulcerated. The polyp is heavily infiltrated by lymphocytes, plasma cells, and macrophages and may contain giant cell granulomas representing a reaction to keratin or cholesterol. Gland-like structures lined by metaplastic cuboidal or columnar ciliated epithelium may be present.

107 Necrotizing External Otitis ("Malignant" Otitis Externa)

Infection of the external auditory canal associated with necrotizing suppurative inflammation which typically spreads to involve adjacent tissues including auricular cartilage and bone.

Pseudomonas aeruginosa and anaerobic organisms are believed to be the major causative agents. The disease occurs mainly in elderly patients and diabetics.

108 Fibro-inflammatory Pseudotumour (Tumefactive Fibro-inflammatory Lesion) (Fig. 161)

A locally destructive lesion composed of fibrovascular tissue admixed with chronic inflammatory cells.

The lesion may contain areas of fibrosis and occasional pockets of neutrophil leucocytes. Atypical fibroblasts with pleomorphic nuclei and prominent nucleoli are occasionally present. Mitoses are scarce. The lesion has poorly defined margins and tends to involve surrounding structures including the orbit. It should be distinguished from infective granulomas (item 109), nodular fasciitis (item 126), aggressive fibromatosis (item 46), fibrous histiocytoma (item 49), malignant fibrous histiocytoma (item 61) and fibrosarcoma (item 60).

109 Infective Granulomas (Figs. 162–169)

A variety of infections give rise to nodular or ulcerative tumour-like lesions in the upper respiratory tract and ear. The lesions usually exhibit infiltration by lymphocytes and plasma cells and may contain granulomas with histiocytes and giant cells. There may also be foci of suppuration, necrosis and pseudoepitheliomatous hyperplasia. The salient features of some of the more common lesions are given below.

Scleroma (Rhinoscleroma) (Figs. 162, 163). Caused by *Klebsiella rhinoscleromatis*, a capsulated gram-negative bacillus. Large nodular tumour-like masses are found in the nasal cavity and less often in other parts of the upper respiratory tract. They contain large macrophages with abundant clear or vacuolated cytoplasm (Mikulicz cells) in which the causative organisms may be identified by the Warthin-Starry staining method or by immunostaining for the *Klebsiella* capsular antigen. There is heavy infiltration by chronic inflammatory cells, mainly plasma cells; there are numerous Russell bodies.

Tuberculosis (Fig. 164). Caused by *Mycobacterium tuberculosis.* The affected tissues contain caseating or non-caseating granulomas with epithelioid histiocytes and Langhans giant cells. Acid fast bacilli are usually demonstrable by the Ziehl-Neelsen method. The lesion occurs most commonly in the larynx in cases of active pulmonary tuberculosis.

Leprosy (Fig. 165). Caused by *Mycobacterium leprae.* The histological picture may be lepromatous, tuberculoid or indeterminate. Lepromatous leprosy is characterized by nodular masses of foamy macrophages (lepra cells) in which large numbers of acid fast bacilli are demonstrable by the modified Ziehl-Neelsen method. Tuberculoid leprosy is characterized by non-caseating granulomas and the indeterminate variant by a non-specific chronic inflammatory reaction; acid fast bacilli are seldom demonstrable in these types.

Rhinosporidiosis (Fig. 166). Caused by the endosporulating fungus *Rhinosporidium seeberi.* The lesions are polypoid and occur principally in the nasal cavity and rarely in the larynx. They are characterized by the presence of thick-walled sporangia measuring 50–350 µm in diameter and containing numerous mucicarminophilic spores. They are associated with a heavy chronic inflammatory reaction with occasional foci of suppuration and foreign body giant cell reaction.

Aspergillosis (Fig. 167). Caused by *Aspergillus fumigatus, Aspergillus niger* and other *Aspergillus* species. The fungi are seen in sections stained with PAS or Gomori methanamine silver as dichotomously branching septate hyphae 6–8 µm wide. Aspergillosis may occur as a non-invasive disease in which a mass of fungal hyphae (fungal ball) is present in a sinus or as an invasive disease, seen more often in immunocompromised patients, associated with destructive inflammation of the sinonasal tissues. The disease may also occur as an allergic aspergillus sinusitis in which the sinuses contain masses of inspissated mucus containing eosinophils, Charcot-Leyden crystals, necrotic cell debris and fungal hyphae; the sinus mucosa shows inflammatory changes without fungal invasion.

Zygomycosis (Mucormycosis). Caused by fungi of the class Zygomycetes and order Mucorales; the most common species causing sinonasal infection are *Rhizopus arrhizus* and *Rhizopus oryzae.* In sections stained with PAS or Gomori methanamine silver the fungi are seen as 10- to 20-µm wide non-septate hyphae, usually branching at right angles. Infection is usually opportunistic and causes rapidly progressive disease in poorly controlled diabetics and immunocompromised patients. The fungus has a tendency to invade blood vessels causing thrombosis; the affected tissues may exhibit coagulative necrosis and haemorrhage.

Candidosis. Caused by *Candida albicans* and other *Candida* species. The condition is usually found in patients suffering from chronic debilitating illnesses or undergoing treatment with corticosteroids or immunosuppressive agents. The lesions show necrosis, suppuration and tuberculoid-type granulomas.

Histoplasmosis (Fig. 168). Caused by *Histoplasma capsulatum.* The capsulated yeast form of the organism, measuring 3–5 µm, is usually found in large numbers within macrophages and giant cells; it is readily identified in sections stained with PAS or Gomori methanamine silver. The lesions, found most commonly in the larynx, are ulcerative and often have raised margins with pseudoepitheliomatous hyperplasia. They are characterized by heavy inflammatory reaction in the early stages of the disease and formation of granulomas in the later stages.

Other Mycoses. Other fungal infections that may occur in the upper respiratory tract include South American blastomycosis *(Blastomyces braziliensis)*, North American blastomycosis *(Blastomyces dermatitidis)*, cryptococcosis *(Cryptococcus neoformans)*, chromomycosis *(Phialophora verrucosa, P. pedrosoi)* and coccidioidomycosis *(Coccidioides immitis)*.

Leishmaniasis (Fig. 169). Caused by *Leishmania braziliensis.* This protozoan parasite, seen in the cytoplasm of histiocytes or extracellularly, measures 1.5–3.0 µm in maximum dimension and has a nucleus and a rod-shaped kinetoplast which stains positively with Giemsa. The kinetoplast is more readily identified in Giemsa-stained smears of exudates or scrapings than in paraffin sections. The lesions, commonly found in the nasal mucosa and facial skin, are markedly destructive and are associated with chronic inflammatory reaction and granuloma formation.

110 Wegener Granulomatosis (Figs. 170, 171)

An immunologically mediated inflammatory disease in which necrotizing angiitis-associated granulomatous lesions occur in the upper respiratory tract and lungs in association with glomerulitis and disseminated small vessel vasculitis.

The lesions in the upper respiratory tract are ulcerative and destructive and occur mainly in the nasal cavity and paranasal sinuses. They are characterized by the presence of geographic necrosis surrounded by palisaded histiocytes, granulomas and scattered giant cells, vasculitis with fibrinoid necrosis or infiltration of vessel walls by inflammatory cells, neutrophilic microabscesses and a mixed inflammatory infiltrate with variable fibrosis. Stains for acid fast bacilli and fungi are negative. There is no cytological atypia. The classic histological features of Wegener granulomatosis are not present in many biopsy specimens. Repeat biopsies and clinical correlations are often essential for early diagnosis. The lesions and symptomatology of Wegener granulomatosis may be restricted to the upper respiratory tract in the early stages of the disease.

111 Foreign Body Granuloma

The presence of exogenous particulate or poorly soluble material in any part of the upper respiratory tract or ear usually results in a foreign body granulomatous reaction. The injection of long-acting prednisolone for the relief of nasal obstruction may produce sinonasal granulomas with a central zone of amorphous basophilic lipid-positive material, sometimes containing birefringent crystals, surrounded by foamy histiocytes and foreign body giant cells. The injection of Teflon into paralysed vocal cords may result in fibrosis and foreign body giant cell reaction; the Teflon particles are birefringent and in H & E stained sections are seen as rounded or irregular foreign bodies with glassy central zones and dark borders.

112 Epidermoid Cholesteatoma (Fig. 172)

A cyst-like lesion of the middle ear cleft that is lined by stratified squamous epithelium and filled with laminated masses of keratin.

The lesion generally occurs as a complication of otitis media and is usually found in the epitympanic recess and the mastoid antrum. It may be associated with chronic inflammatory reaction, haemorrhage, granulomatous reaction to keratin or cholesterol and pressure necrosis of adjacent bone.

113 Cholesterol Granuloma (Fig.173)

A granulomatous lesion containing cholesterol crystals.

This lesion is a sequel of otitis media or haemorrhage into the tympanic cavity. It may also occur in association with cholesteatoma (item 112). In routinely processed sections the cholesterol crystals, derived from the breakdown of blood and inflammatory exudate, are seen as empty clefts surrounded and engulfed by multinucleated foreign body giant cells in a background of fibrous granulation tissue; chronic inflammatory changes and haemosiderin deposits are common.

114 "Myospherulosis" (Spherulocystic Disease)

This lesion is characterized by the presence of cyst-like spaces lined by flattened histiocytes and containing clusters of brownish spherules resembling fungi lying loosely or within sacs formed by thin refractile membranes. The brownish spherules do not stain with PAS or Gomori methanamine silver and their morphology does not correspond with any known fungus. They are found within fibrous granulation tissue which may show a foreign body reaction. The lesion is usually found in patients who have had previous operations. It is now recognized that the spherules are extravasated red cells that have been altered by interaction with traumatised fat or petrolatum-based ointments and gauzes used in surgical procedures.

115 Seborrhoeic Keratosis (Basal Cell Papilloma) (Fig.174)

A skin lesion characterized by a sharply defined area of epidermal thickening consisting mainly of basaloid cells with variable squamous differentiation and foci of abrupt keratinization.

The entire lesion is raised above the level of the marginal skin. The lesion frequently exhibits hyperkeratosis and papillomatosis; it often contains melanocytes and may be heavily pigmented.

116 Verruca Vulgaris

Warty hyperplasia of squamous epithelium associated with human papilloma virus infection.

The squamous epithelium typically shows papillomatosis, acanthosis and hyperkeratosis with parakeratosis. It has a prominent granular layer with cells containing large keratohyaline granules and cells with pyknotic nuclei surrounded by a halo of clear cytoplasm (koilocytes) in the superficial layers. The rete ridges at the periphery of the lesion are usually bent inwards towards the centre.

117 Pseudoepitheliomatous Hyperplasia (Figs. 95, 175)

A reactive or reparative overgrowth of squamous epithelium that histologically mimics carcinoma.

The epithelium is well differentiated and does not exhibit any cytological evidence of malignancy. The rete ridges are elongated and when sectioned tangentially appear as anastomosing epithelial strands and nests separated from the surface simulating invasion. The stroma is usually infiltrated by chronic inflammatory cells. This reaction may occur at sites of injury or chronic irritation, in chronic infective or ulcerative lesions and in association with granular cell tumour (item 58). The absence of cytologic atypia and the clinical setting are helpful in distinguishing the lesion from squamous cell carcinoma.

118 Keratoacanthoma (Fig. 176)

This lesion is seen clinically as a nodular dome-shaped skin lesion with a central keratin-filled crater; it grows rapidly to reach a maximum size (1–2.5 cm) within 1–2 months and involutes spontaneously within 4–6 months. Histologically the lesion appears as a raised hemispherical mass in the dermis composed of a central plug of keratin surrounded by nests and columns of squamous epithelium. There is limited pushing infiltration at the outer margin which seldom extends below the level of the sweat glands. A chronic inflammatory reaction is typically present at the periphery. The epidermis covering the lesion dips into the sides of the central keratin-filled crater. The lesion may exhibit cytologic atypia, dyskeratosis and mitotic activity. It is distinguished from squamous cell carcinoma by its clinical features and by its overall architecture; the latter however may not be evident in biopsies that do not include the central crater, base and margins of the lesion.

119 Squamous Cell Hyperplasia (Fig. 177)

A lesion in which the squamous epithelium shows an increase in cells and in cell layers (acanthosis) without cellular atypia or loss of normal stratification.

Squamous cell hyperplasia is common in laryngeal oedema, polyps and in metaplastic squamous epithelium adjacent to the true vocal cords. It is a reactive process which should not, particularly when seen in metaplastic squamous epithelium, be misinterpreted as dysplasia (item 18). The lesion is often associated with keratosis (item 120).

120 Keratosis (Fig. 178)

In keratosis of the larynx the more superficial epithelial layers show keratinization with formation of squames or keratohyaline granules; the surface is covered by keratin or parakeratin. Laryngeal keratosis is often associated with squamous cell hyperplasia (item 119) and dysplasia (item 18).

121 Keratosis Obturans

A form of squamous cell hyperplasia and hyperkeratosis in which there is accumulation of a large amount of desquamated keratin in the external auditory canal.

The presence of a mass of keratin in the auditory meatus may lead to inflammatory reaction and pressure necrosis of bone. The condition is often bilateral.

122 Necrotizing Sialometaplasia (Fig. 179)

Squamous metaplasia of the ducts and acini of seromucinous glands following necrosis or ulceration.

The lesion may follow ischaemia or trauma and resolves spontaneously. It is often ulcerated and may be accompanied by pseudoepitheliomatous hyperplasia, inflammatory reaction and mucus extravasation. The metaplastic squamous epithelium usually fills the ducts and acini, forming solid nests that may simulate carcinoma. The benign cytological features and preservation of lobular architecture distinguish the lesion from squamous cell carcinoma and mucoepidermoid carcinoma.

123 Adenomatoid Hyperplasia

In the upper respiratory tract this lesion occurs as a nodular mass composed of lobules of hyperplastic or hypertrophied seromucinous glands comprising secretory and ductal elements. The stroma may show extravasated mucin and mild inflammatory changes. The mucosal surface is usually unremarkable.

124 Oncocytic Metaplasia and Hyperplasia (Figs. 180, 181)

Replacement of ducts and acini of seromucinous glands by cells with abundant brightly eosinophilic granular cytoplasm (oncocytes).

Oncocytes have small hyperchromatic nuclei and their cytoplasm is packed with mitochondria as shown by positive staining with PTAH and, more definitively, by electron microscopy. Oncocytic metaplasia is characteristically patchy in distribution. The partial involvement of glandular units and the presence of ducts within the lesion are helpful in distinguishing the lesion from oncocytoma (item 9). The oncocytic lesion in the larynx to which the term *oncocytic papillary cystadenoma* has been applied has a cystic structure with papillary infoldings lined by bilayered oncocytic epithelium.

125 Keloid

An overgrowth of dermal scar tissue containing broad eosinophilic bands of hyalinized collagen.

The lesion usually follows some form of injury and represents a slowly progressive but limited overgrowth of scar tissue. A few fibroblasts and some mucoid ground substance are usually present between the collagen bundles. Long-standing cases may exhibit calcification or osseous metaplasia. The lesion has a tendency to recur after removal.

126 Nodular Fasciitis (Pseudosarcomatous Fasciitis) (Fig. 182)

A benign reparative self-limited proliferation of fibroblast-like cells.

In the upper respiratory tract this lesion usually occurs in the submucosal soft tissues with attachment to fascia. The lesion is composed of plump spindle or stellate cells resembling fibroblasts or myofibroblasts. The cells are arranged loosely in curved fascicles in an oedematous or myxoid matrix giving a tissue culture-like appearance. Capillaries are present throughout the lesion and are especially prominent at the periphery where they tend to be radially arranged. Typical mitoses are common and may be numerous. The lesion frequently contains bands of collagen, extravasated red cells, lymphocytes, foamy macrophages and a few giant cells. There may be pools of acid mucopolysaccharide-rich fluid. The lesion usually measures less than 3 cm in diameter and may be partially circumscribed but is not encapsulated. It grows very rapidly and may regress spontaneously within weeks or months.

127 Granuloma Pyogenicum (Lobular Capillary Haemangioma) (Figs. 183, 184)

A rapidly growing lobular proliferation of capillaries.

The lesion is usually exophytic and dome-shaped. It consists of lobules of capillaries separated by loose connective tissue stroma that is often infiltrated by inflammatory cells. Feeder arteries and small post-capillary venules may be identified in favourably oriented sections. Mitoses are present in both capillary endothelium and stroma. The epithelium covering the lesion is usually atrophic and ulcerated and may show hyperplastic changes at the margins with the formation of a collarette at the base. The lesion probably represents a vascular reaction to injury. It grows rapidly and usually regresses spontaneously with fibrosis within weeks or months. Histological differentiation between granuloma pyogenicum and haemangioma (item 53) can be difficult.

128 Intubation Granuloma/Contact Ulcer (Figs. 185, 186)

These lesions occur as hemispherical masses of highly vascular granulation tissue situated at the posterior ends of the vocal cords over the arytenoid cartilages. They consist mainly of capillary blood vessels arranged radially from the base to a fibrin-coated surface. Fibroblasts and inflammatory cells are present between the capillaries. The marginal epithelium may show pseudoepitheliomatous hyperplasia. The lesion occurring as a complication of endotracheal intubation is found over the vocal processes of the arytenoid cartilages. The lesion referred to as "contact ulcer", variously attributed to injury caused by violent coughing or the action of aspirated oronasal or gastric secretions, may be found over any part of the arytenoids.

129 Elastic Cartilage Metaplasia (Chondroid Metaplasia)

This lesion occurs as a nodule of elastic cartilage in the connective tissue of the vestibular fold or true vocal cord without attachment to laryngeal cartilage. It represents a metaplastic process which commences with the formation of a mucopolysaccharide-rich myxoid nodule. The fully developed lesion is characterized by the presence of large polygonal cells with clear cytoplasm resembling chondrocytes. The lesion is small and frequently bilateral. It should be distinguished from chondroid neoplasms.

130 Tracheopathia Osteochondroplastica (Fig. 187)

A lesion of the trachea characterized by the formation of multiple submucosal nodules composed of metaplastic calcified cartilage and lamellar bone.

131 Chondrodermatitis Nodularis Helicis (Fig. 188)

A chronic nodular lesion of the external ear associated with degenerative and inflammatory changes involving skin, soft tissues and cartilage.

   The epithelium over the lesion is often ulcerated and covered by encrusted necrotic debris; the ulcer margins may show pseudoepitheliomatous hyperplasia and hyperkeratosis. In the subepithelial connective tissues there are areas of fibrinoid material surrounded by granulation tissue and inflammatory cell infiltrates involving the perichondrium. The underlying cartilage may show degenerative changes with formation of cysts or cleft-like spaces.

132 Relapsing Polychondritis (Fig. 189)

An autoimmune disorder characterized by progressive degenerative and inflammatory changes affecting the articular, auricular, nasal and laryngotracheal cartilages.

   In the early stages of the disease there is some eosinophilia of the ground substance of the affected cartilages associated with pyknosis and dissolution of the chondroid cells. This is followed by infiltration by acute and chronic inflammatory cells, formation of granulation tissue, fibrosis and calcification. The disease runs a chronic course with remissions and recurrences; it may be associated with other autoimmune disorders.

133 Cystic Chondromalacia (Enchondral Pseudocyst) of the Auricle (Fig. 190)

A degenerative disease of auricular cartilage associated with the formation of pseudocysts.

The pseudocysts are lined by granulation tissue and/or cartilage. Degenerative and proliferative changes may be present, but there is no cytologic atypia. There may be foci of calcification and ossification. Inflammatory changes are minimal. The lesion occurs within the auricular cartilage and not in a perichondrial location and does not involve overlying skin as in chondrodermatitis nodularis helicis (item 131). It is usually painless and is not associated with systemic symptoms or involvement of other cartilages as in relapsing polychondritis (item 132).

134 Tympanosclerosis (Fig. 191)

The formation of dense hyalinized fibrous tissue in the tympanic membrane and middle ear mucosa.

The hyalinized fibrous tissue undergoes patchy calcification; ossification is common. The lesion is a complication of chronic otitis media and may lead to fixation of the ossicles.

135 Fibrous Dysplasia (Fig. 192)

A self-limiting non-encapsulated lesion characterized by replacement of normal bone by cellular fibrous connective tissue containing irregular trabeculae of immature non-lamellar metaplastic bone.

Cellular fibrous tissue predominates in early lesions and the amount of bone increases with the stage of development. The osseous component typically occurs as irregularly curved trabeculae of woven bone without osteoblastic rimming but spicules of lamellar bone rimmed by osteoblasts are sometimes present, especially in recurrent lesions. Cystic changes, macrophages and giant cells may be present. The lesion is presumably developmental and is usually found in young subjects. The maxilla is the most frequently involved craniofacial bone, followed by the mandible. The distinction from ossifying fibroma (item 75) can be difficult in some cases. The term *benign fibro-osseous lesion* is applied to cases with overlapping histological features.

136 Giant Cell Reparative Granuloma (Fig. 193)

A reactive lesion consisting of cellular fibrous tissue containing foci of haemorrhage and aggregates of multinucleated osteoclast-like giant cells.

The lesion occurs more frequently in children and young adults. It may be central (intra-osseous) or peripheral (periosteal). The fibrous component has a loose texture and usually contains numerous capillaries, haemosiderin deposits and chronic inflammatory cells. Mitoses are common. The multinucleated giant cells are generally smaller and more irregular than those in giant cell tumour of bone (item 76); they exhibit benign cytological features and are usually found in relation to capillaries and foci of haemorrhage. Metaplastic woven bone may be found within septa of mature fibrous tissue that traverse the lesion. The bland cytologic features and the uneven distribution of the giant cells are helpful in distinguishing the lesion from the true giant cell tumour which is rare in the jaws. The bone lesions of hyperparathyroidism ("brown tumour") and cherubism are histologically indistinguishable from giant cell reparative granuloma and should be excluded on the basis of clinical and biochemical findings.

137 Aneurysmal Bone Cyst

A bone lesion characterized by large vascular channels or blood-filled spaces separated by fibrous septa that may contain slivers of bone or osteoid.

Clusters of osteoclast-type giant cells and haemosiderin-containing macrophages are usually present. Aneurysmal bone cyst frequently contains solid areas with histological features similar to giant cell reparative granuloma (item 136).

138 Lymphoid Hyperplasia (Fig. 194)

The nasopharyngeal mucosa contains abundant lymphoid tissue which forms masses with germinal centres in the lateral wall ("tubal tonsil") and upper posterior wall ("pharyngeal tonsil"). These may undergo reactive lymphoid hyperplasia and present as tumour-like swellings.

139 Plasma Cell Granuloma

A chronic inflammatory lesion with heavy plasma cell infiltration.

The lesion is not associated with abnormalities of protein metabolism or bone marrow involvement. It usually occurs in the paranasal sinus mucosa in association with severe chronic sinusitis; lymph follicles are often present. The lesion may be distinguished from extramedullary plasmacytoma (item 82) by the maturity of the plasma cells, presence of Russell bodies, admixture with chronic inflammatory cells and, more definitively, by stains for immunoglobulins which demonstrate a polyclonal plasma cell population.

140 Malakoplakia (Fig. 195)

A chronic inflammatory lesion characterized by the presence of macrophages containing diastase-resistant, PAS-positive granules (von Hansemann macrophages) and rounded concretions with a laminated structure (Michaelis-Gutmann bodies).

The macrophages are usually admixed with lymphocytes, plasma cells and neutrophils. The Michaelis-Gutmann bodies often stain positively for calcium and iron and are found within the macrophages or extracellularly. The condition probably represents an abnormal macrophage response to phagocytosed *Escherichia coli* or other micro-organisms. The lesion may resemble granular cell tumour (item 58) from which it is distinguished by the presence of the characteristic Michaelis-Gutmann bodies.

141 Langerhans Cell Histiocytosis (Histiocytosis X) (Fig. 196)

A solitary or multifocal proliferation of histiocytes with the morphological, ultrastructural and immunocytologic characteristics of Langerhans cells.

This category includes *eosinophilic granuloma* which is an indolent lesion usually restricted to a single bone, *Hand-Schuller-Christian disease* in which chronic lesions are present in multiple bones and other tissues and *Letterer-Siwe disease* which is a rapidly progressive systemic form of histiocytosis which usually occurs in infancy. Some cases of Letterer-Siwe disease may represent a malignant form of histiocytosis.

The lesions are composed of a meshwork of histiocytes which have indented or grooved nuclei, inconspicuous nucleoli, sharply defined nuclear membranes and pale or eosinophilic cytoplasm that is often finely vacuolated. A few mitoses may be present. Aggregates of eosinophil leucocytes are present among the histiocytes. Haemorrhage, necrosis, foamy macrophages, giant cells and other inflammatory cells are frequently present. Langerhans histiocytes are immunoreactive for CD-1 and S-100 protein and may be specifically identified by electron microscopy which reveals characteristic rod-shaped granules (Birbeck granules).

142 Angiolymphoid Hyperplasia with Eosinophilia (Epithelioid Haemangioma, Histiocytoid Haemangioma)
(Fig. 197)

The lesions in this disease usually occur as one or more papules or nodules in the face and scalp, especially around the ear, involving the dermis and superficial subcutaneous tissue. They are characterized by vascular proliferation and infiltrates of lymphocytes and eosinophils. There is marked proliferation of capillaries, often around arteries or veins. The endothelium lining the vessels usually exhibits epithelioid of histiocytoid features; uncanalized or poorly canalized cords or nests of such cells may also be present. The endothelial cells have hyperchromatic nuclei and eosinophilic cytoplasm which often contains vacuoles. Mitoses may be present. There are infiltrates of lymphocytes and eosinophils, but these are seldom as prominent as those in Kimura disease (item 143). The question of whether angiolymphoid hyperplasia with eosinophilia represents a vascular neoplasm or a reactive phenomenon is not settled.

143 Kimura Disease (Fig. 198)

The lesions in this disease usually occur as large poorly defined subcutaneous or deep-seated soft tissue masses, especially in the periauricular region, cheek and submandibular region; they may involve salivary gland and striated muscle. They exhibit heavy infiltration by eosinophils and marked lymphoid hyperplasia with formation of germinal centres. The eosinophils may coalesce to form microabscesses and may extend into the germinal centres causing folliculolysis. Fibrosis may be prominent. Some vascular proliferation may be present, and the endothelial cells may appear swollen, but they do not exhibit epithelioid of histiocytoid features or form uncanalized cords as in angiolymphoid hyperplasia with eosinophilia (item 142).

The lesions have a tendency to recur and usually persist for several years. The regional lymph nodes are often enlarged and exhibit vascular proliferation and eosinophilic infiltration.

144 Rosai-Dorfman Disease (Sinus Histiocytosis with Massive Lymphadenopathy) (Fig. 199)

The lesions in the upper respiratory tract are characterized by infiltrates of the same type of atypical histiocyte as found in the subcapsular and medullary sinuses of lymph nodes in the classical nodal form of the disease. These cells have a large vesicular nucleus with a prominent nucleolus and abundant weakly staining eosinophilic cytoplasm that is often foamy and may contain lipid. The presence of lymphocytes in the cytoplasm of some of these cells following lymphophagocytosis or emperipolesis is a characteristic feature of this disease. Mitoses are rare. By immunostaining the histiocytes are positive for S-100 protein and negative for CD-1; by electron microscopy they lack Birbeck granules.

In the upper respiratory tract the histiocytes occur in irregular sheets or aggregates surrounded by lymphocytes and plasma cells; Russell bodies are usually prominent. Fibrosis and xanthomatous reaction are generally more marked and lymphophagocytosis less prominent than in the nodal lesions. The disease has a prolonged clinical course but sometimes regresses quickly and spontaneously. It should be distinguished from the histiocytic lymphomas (item 84), Langerhans cell histiocytosis (item 141), infective granulomas (item 109), and the storage diseases.

145 Amyloid Deposits (Fig. 200)

Amyloid deposition may occur in any part of the upper respiratory tract as an isolated phenomenon or as part of systemic amyloidosis. Localized amyloid deposits occur most commonly in the larynx. Amyloid deposition usually begins in the walls of blood vessels and the basal lamina of seromucous glands and progresses to form nodular masses. In routinely stained sections amyloid appears as pale eosinophilic hyaline material and is frequently associated with a foreign body giant cell reaction. The staining reactions and ultrastructural characteristics of amyloid in this location are similar to those in other parts of the body.

146 Gouty Tophi

Deposits of urates in the capsules of joints, cartilages and soft tissues.

Deposits of urates may occur in the cartilage of the external ear in cases of gout; very rarely they may also occur in the vocal cord and laryngeal cartilages. In smears of gouty discharges and in sections of fresh-frozen or alcohol-fixed tissues the urates are seen as sheaves of fine brownish needle-shaped birefringent crystals which stain positively with the De Galantha silver nitrate and Gomori hexamine-silver techniques. In sections of tissues fixed in aqueous formaldehyde solutions the gouty tophi are seen as pale amorphous masses surrounded by foreign body giant cells, histiocytes and fibrous tissue.

147 Lipoid Proteinosis

An inherited disorder characterized by the presence of widespread nodules, plaques and ulcerated lesions in the skin and mucous membranes associated with deposits of lipid and glycoproteins in the connective tissues.

Amorphous eosinophilic hyaline deposits of diastase-resistant PAS-positive material containing lipid droplets occur around capillary walls and adjacent connective tissues. In the upper respiratory tract the lesions occur most frequently in the larynx.

Subject Index

Unless otherwise stated, all the preparations shown in the photomicrographs reproduced on the following pages were stained with haematoxylin-eosin.

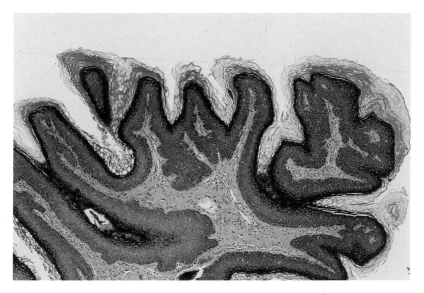

Fig. 1. *Squamous cell papilloma,* pinna. Fronds of well-differentiated keratinizing stratified squamous epithelium with cores of fibrous stroma

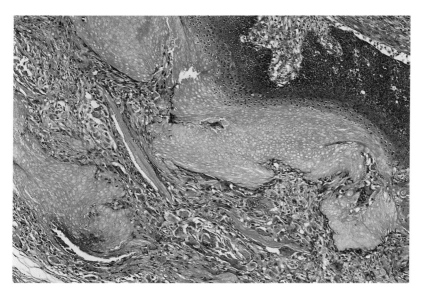

Fig. 2. *Pilomatrixoma,* pinna. Islands of basophilic cells and "ghost" cells with non-staining nuclei. Giant cell reaction to keratin

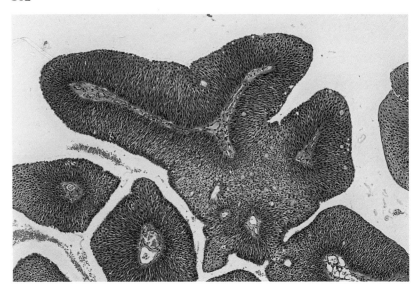

Fig. 3. *Exophytic papilloma,* nasal septum. Fronds of nasal respiratory-type epithelium with squamoid features

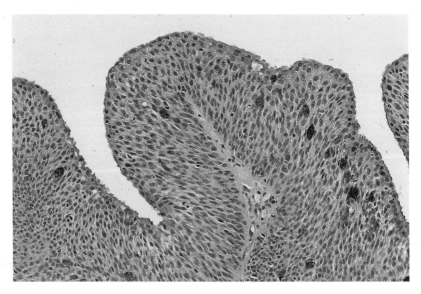

Fig. 4. *Exophytic papilloma,* nasal septum. Mucin-secreting cells within stratified epithelium. Same case as Fig. 3. Mucicarmine

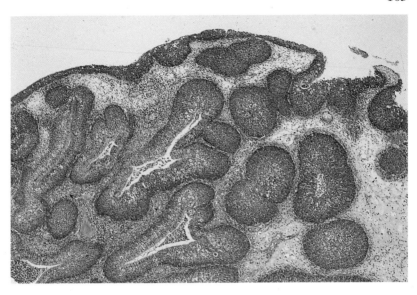

Fig. 5. *Inverted papilloma,* lateral nasal wall. Invaginations of sinonasal epithelium

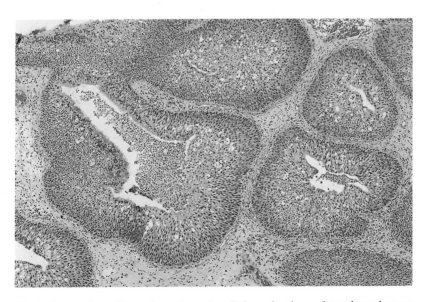

Fig. 6. *Inverted papilloma,* lateral nasal wall. Invaginations of nasal respiratory epithelium containing inflammatory cells

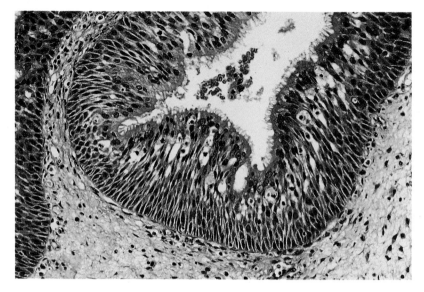

Fig. 7. *Inverted papilloma,* maxillary sinus. Crypts lined by pseudostratified ciliated epithelium

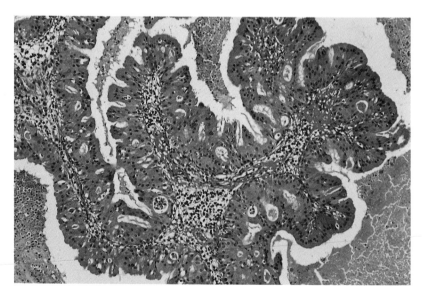

Fig. 8. *Columnar cell papilloma,* maxillary sinus. Papillary eversions covered by columnar epithelium with oncocytic features. Intraepithelial microcysts

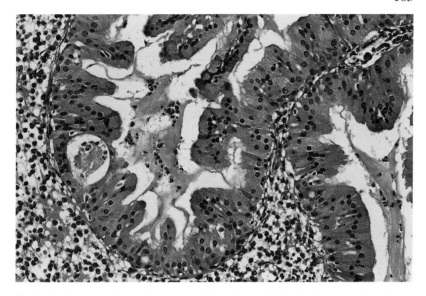

Fig. 9. *Columnar cell papilloma,* maxillary sinus. Epithelial invaginations lined by columnar cells with oncocytic features. Intraepithelial mucin-filled cysts and microabscesses

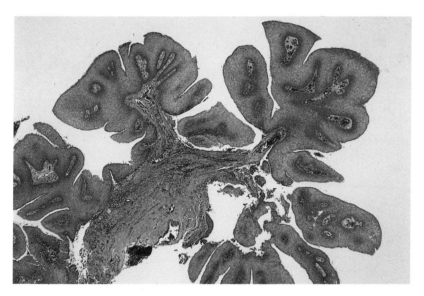

Fig. 10. *Laryngeal papilloma.* Fronds of well-differentiated stratified squamous epithelium

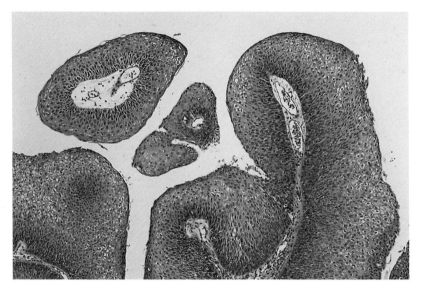

Fig. 11. *Laryngeal papilloma, non-keratinizing.* Papillary processes covered by non-keratinizing stratified squamous epithelium. Fibrovascular stroma

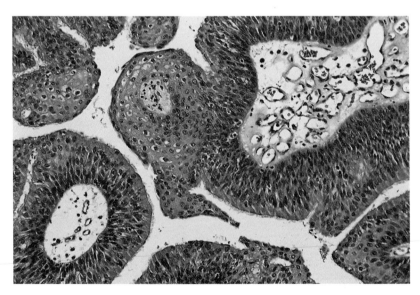

Fig. 12. *Laryngeal papilloma, non-keratinizing.* Papillary processes covered by ciliated respiratory-type epithelium and non-keratinizing stratified squamous epithelium. Fibrovascular stroma

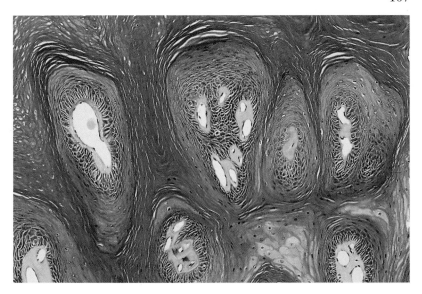

Fig. 13. *Laryngeal papilloma, keratinizing.* Mass of keratin separating papillary processes covered by keratinizing squamous epithelium

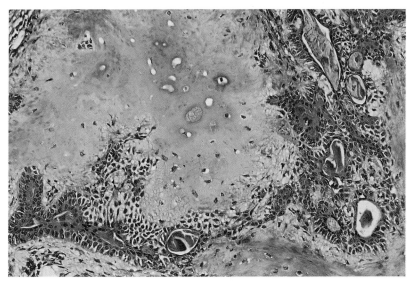

Fig. 14. *Pleomorphic adenoma,* nasal septum. Luminal-type epithelial cells, myoepithelial cells and chondroid tissue

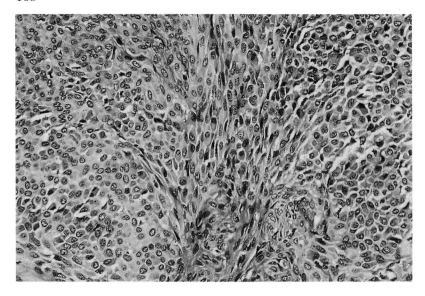

Fig. 15. *Myoepithelioma, lateral nasal wall.* Closely packed spindle-shaped cells and plasmacytoid or hyaline cells

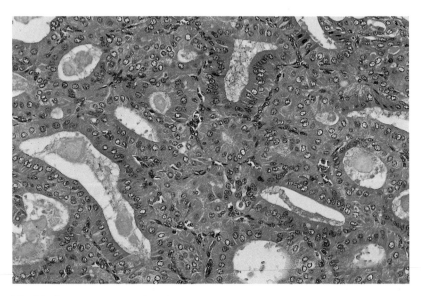

Fig. 16. *Oncocytoma,* nasal cavity. Glandular structures, lined by columnar cells with abundant eosinophilic cytoplasm

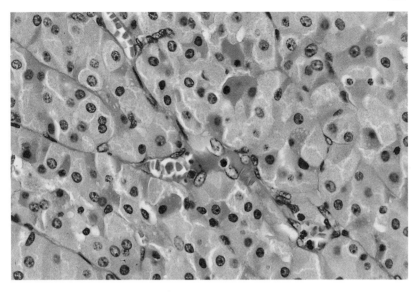

Fig. 17. *Oncocytoma,* nasal cavity. Compact sheets of pale and dark cells with regular nuclei and abundant eosinophilic cytoplasm

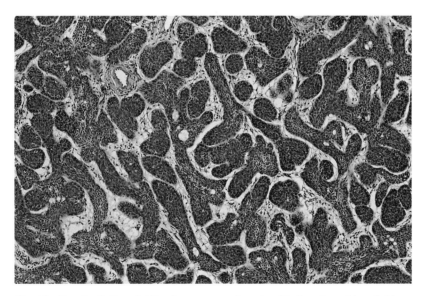

Fig. 18. *Basal cell (basaloid) adenoma,* nasal cavity. Trabeculae of basaloid tumour cells with peripheral palisading

110

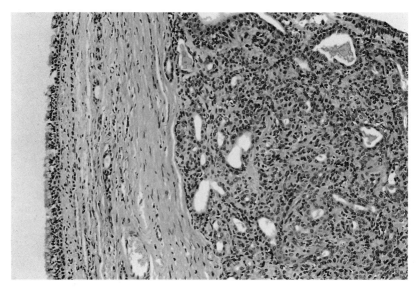

Fig. 19. *Basal cell (basaloid) adenoma,* nasal cavity. Encapsulated tumour with trabecular-tubular structure

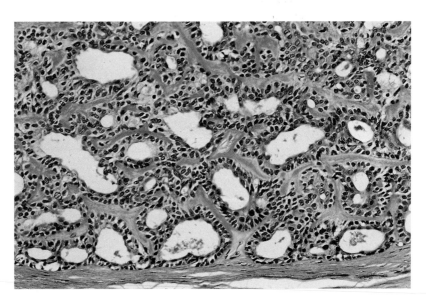

Fig. 20. *Basal cell (basaloid) adenoma,* nasal cavity. Tubules lined by bilayered basaloid and luminal-type epithelium. Same case as Fig. 19

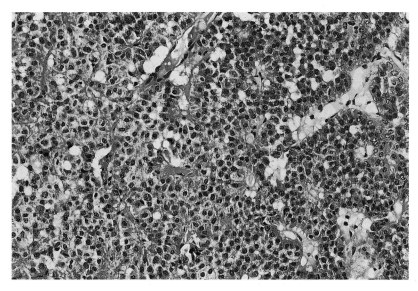

Fig. 21. *Ectopic pituitary adenoma,* roof of nasopharynx. Sheets of polyhedral pituitary-type cells. Vascular stroma

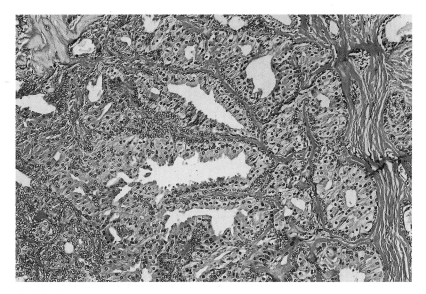

Fig. 22. *Ceruminous adenoma,* external auditory meatus. Glandular structures lined by bilayered epithelium – an inner layer of apocrine epithelium with apical snouts and an outer layer of myoepithelial cells

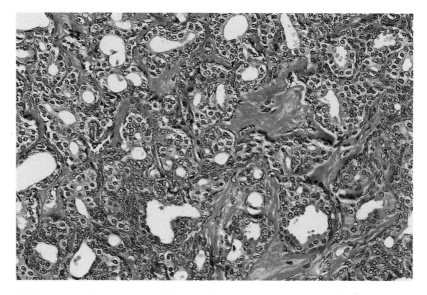

Fig. 23. *Ceruminous adenoma,* external auditory meatus. Glandular structures lined by bilayered epithelium. Fibrous stroma

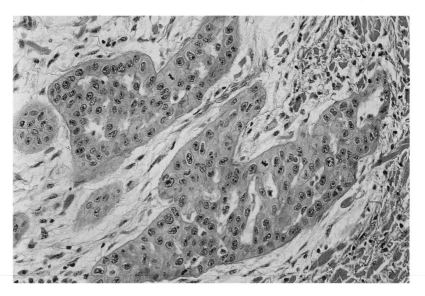

Fig. 24. *Ceruminous adenocarcinoma,* external auditory meatus. Sheets of cells with poorly formed glandular lumina, mitoses and stromal invasion

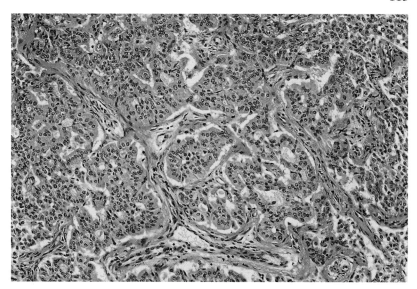

Fig. 25. *Adenoma of middle ear.* Glandular structures lined by a single layer of uniform cuboidal and low columnar cells. Back-to-back pattern

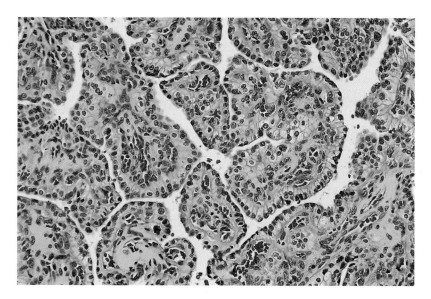

Fig. 26. *Papillary adenoma,* inner ear. Papillary structures covered by cuboidal epithelial cells

114

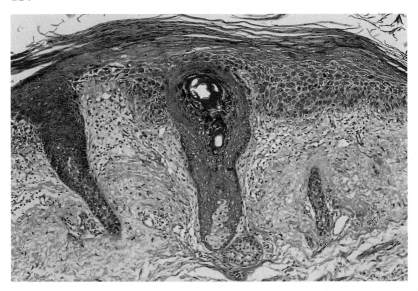

Fig. 27. Solar keratosis, pinna. Epidermal dysplasia with moderate nuclear atypia, mitotic activity and keratosis. Dermal elastosis

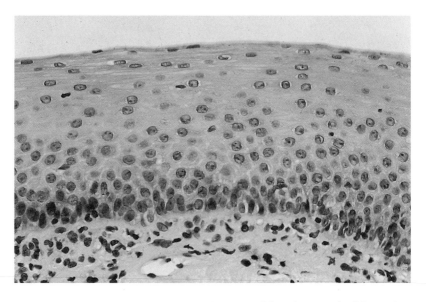

Fig. 28. *Squamous cell dysplasia, mild,* larynx. Mild nuclear atypia. Maturation and stratification of upper layers

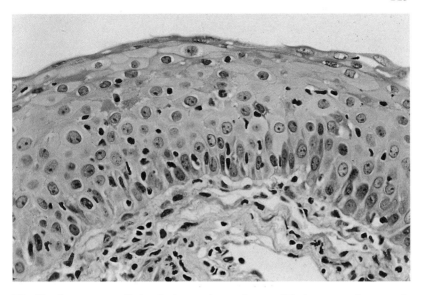

Fig. 29. *Squamous cell dysplasia, moderate,* larynx. Moderate nuclear atypia with prominent nucleoli. Stratification of upper layers

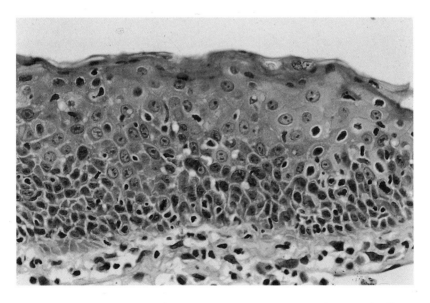

Fig. 30. *Squamous cell dysplasia, severe,* larynx. Severe nuclear atypia. Some maturation and stratification of the most superficial layers. Several mitoses

116

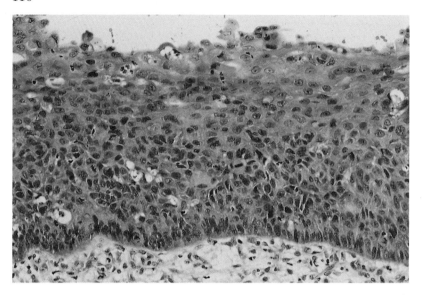

Fig. 31. *Carcinoma in situ,* larynx. Severe nuclear atypia and loss of cell stratification involving full epithelial thickness. Minimal keratinization. Several mitoses

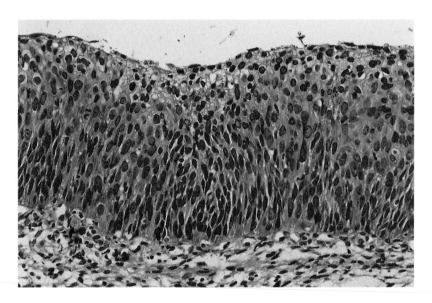

Fig. 32. *Carcinoma in situ,* larynx. Severe nuclear atypia and loss of cell stratification involving full epithelial thickness. Closely packed non-keratinizing cells with hyperchromatic nuclei. Several mitoses, some abnormal, in upper layers

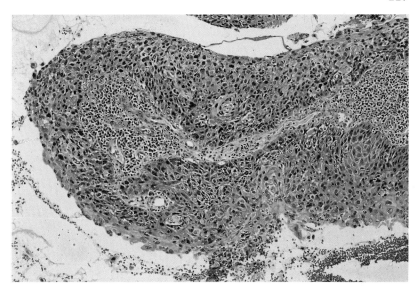

Fig. 33. *Papillary carcinoma in situ,* hypopharynx. Papillary structure covered by stratified squamous epithelium with cytologic features of malignancy. Basement membrane intact

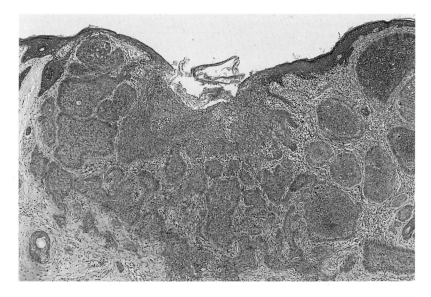

Fig. 34. *Basal cell carcinoma,* pinna. Downgrowths of compact masses of uniform basal-type cells with peripheral palisading

118

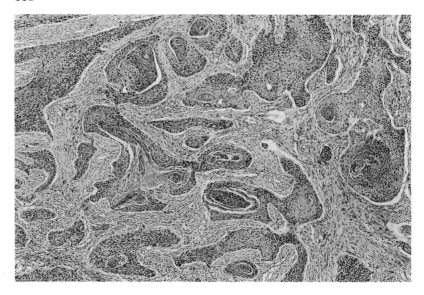

Fig. 35. *Squamous cell carcinoma,* larynx. Infiltrating nests of keratinizing squamous cell carcinoma

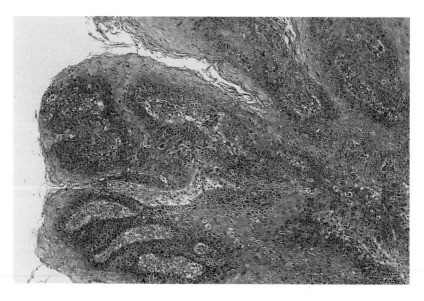

Fig. 36. *Papillary squamous cell carcinoma,* larynx. Squamous cell carcinoma composed mainly of exophytic papillary structures covered by epithelium showing severe nuclear atypia and high mitotic activity

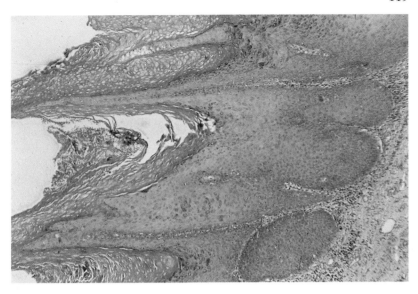

Fig. 37. *Verrucous squamous cell carcinoma,* larynx. Vertical folds of well-differentiated stratified squamous epithelium covered by keratin. Bland cytologic features

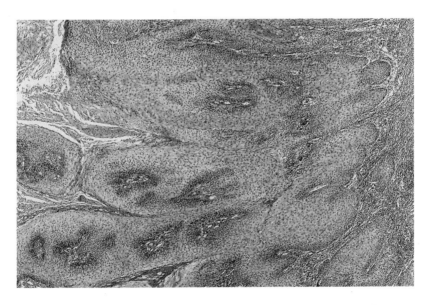

Fig. 38. *Verrucous squamous cell carcinoma,* larynx. Exophytic papillary tumour composed of stratified squamous epithelium with bland cytologic features. Rete pegs elongated and bulbous

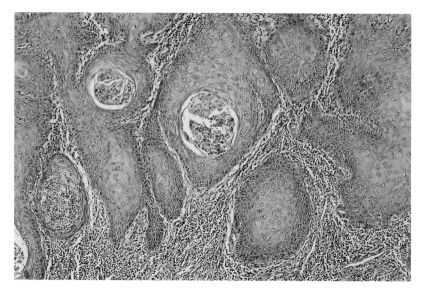

Fig. 39. *Verrucous squamous cell carcinoma,* larynx. Deep portion of tumour showing bulbous "pushing" downgrowths, some containing microabscesses, associated with chronic inflammatory reaction

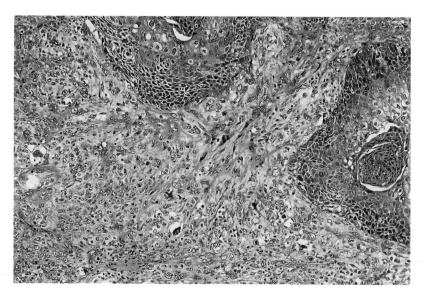

Fig. 40. *Spindle cell carcinoma,* hypopharynx. Bimorphic tumour comprising a moderately differentiated keratinizing squamous cell carcinoma and a sarcoma-like pleomorphic spindle-cell component

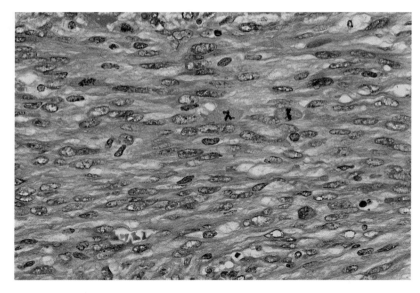

Fig. 41. *Spindle cell carcinoma,* larynx. Squamous cell carcinoma with pseudo-sarcomatous spindle-cell structure

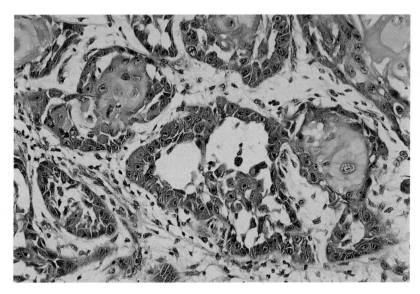

Fig. 42. *Adenoid squamous cell carcinoma,* pinna. Squamous cell carcinoma with acantholysis and formation of pseudoglandular spaces

122

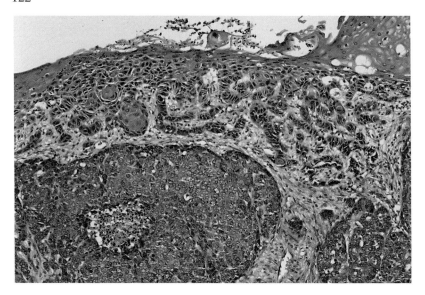

Fig. 43. *Basaloid squamous cell carcinoma.* Bimorphic carcinoma with mass of closely packed basaloid tumour cells with central necrosis and a superficial component of squamous cell carcinoma

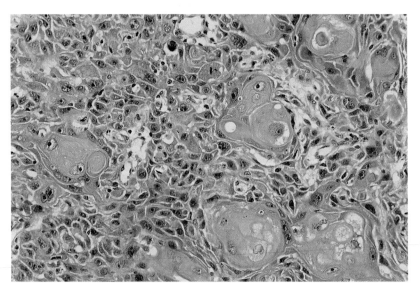

Fig. 44. *Sinonasal carcinoma, squamous cell.* Keratinizing tumour cells with intercellular bridges

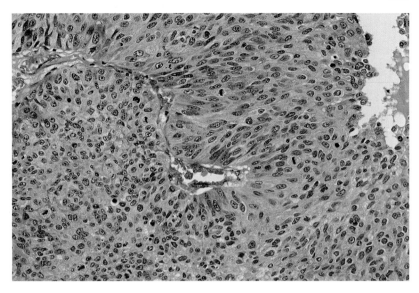

Fig. 45. *Sinonasal carcinoma, cylindrical cell.* Non-keratinizing tumour cells of respiratory epithelial type. Numerous mitoses

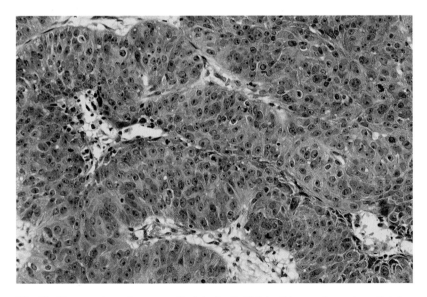

Fig. 46. *Sinonasal carcinoma, cylindrical cell.* Thick ribbons of non-keratinizing tumour cells

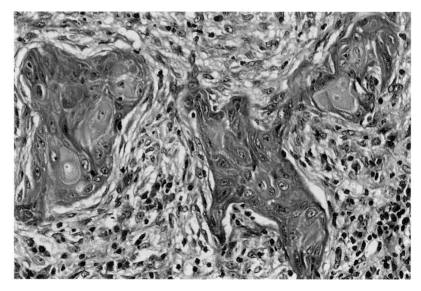

Fig. 47. *Nasopharyngeal carcinoma, squamous cell.* Well-differentiated squamous cell carcinoma with keratinization and intercellular bridges

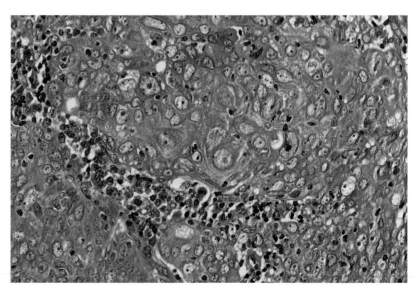

Fig. 48. *Nasopharyngeal carcinoma, squamous cell.* Moderately differentiated squamous cell carcinoma with focal keratinization

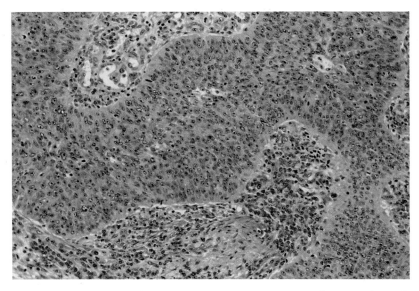

Fig. 49. *Nasopharyngeal carcinoma, non-keratinizing, differentiated.* Well-defined plexiform masses of non-keratinizing tumour cells

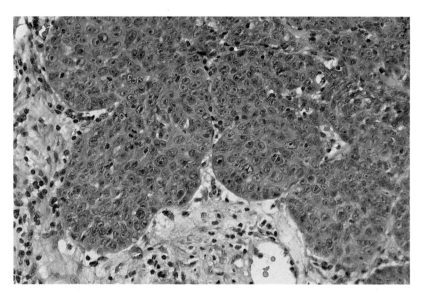

Fig. 50. *Nasopharyngeal carcinoma, non-keratinizing, differentiated.* Well-defined masses of closely packed non-keratinizing tumour cells

126

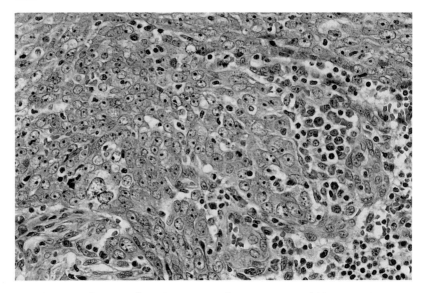

Fig. 51. *Nasopharyngeal carcinoma, non-keratinizing, undifferentiated.* Syncytial masses of undifferentiated tumour cells with vesicular nuclei and prominent nucleoli. Lymphocytes and plasma cells in stroma

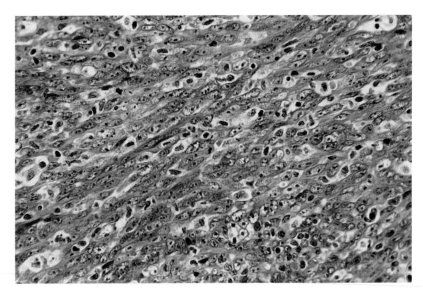

Fig. 52. *Nasopharyngeal carcinoma, non-keratinizing, undifferentiated.* Undifferentiated carcinoma with spindle-cell structure

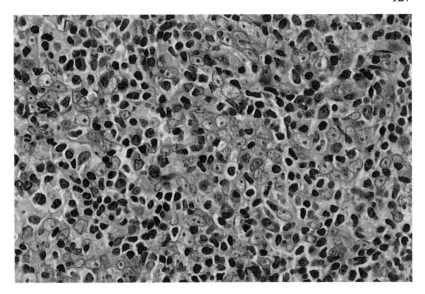

Fig. 53. *Nasopharyngeal carcinoma, non-keratinizing, undifferentiated.* Undifferentiated carcinoma heavily admixed with lymphocytes and plasma cells – lymphoepithelial carcinoma

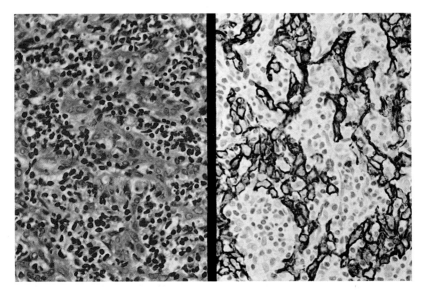

Fig. 54. *Nasopharyngeal carcinoma, non-keratinizing, undifferentiated.* Undifferentiated carcinoma with lymphoid stroma – lymphoepithelial carcinoma. H & E/anti-keratin, wide spectrum

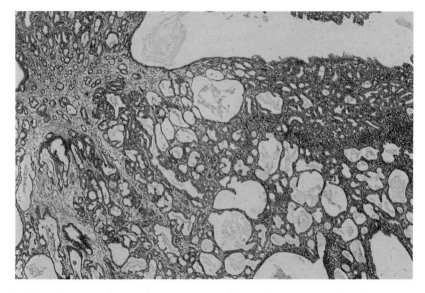

Fig. 55. *Adenocarcinoma, low grade,* nasopharynx. Non-encapsulated glandular tumour with bland cytologic features

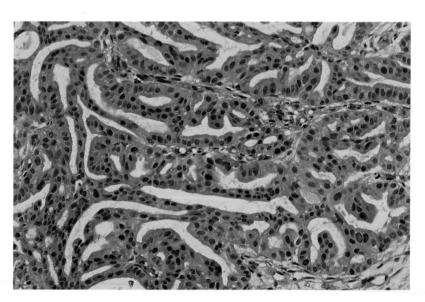

Fig. 56. *Adenocarcinoma, low grade,* nasal cavity. Well-differentiated tubular-glandular structures with back-to-back pattern

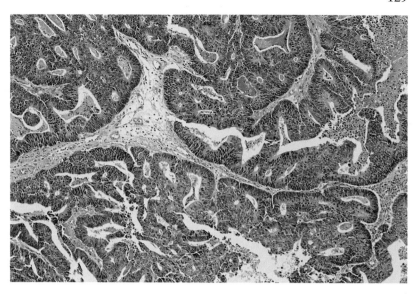

Fig. 57. *Adenocarcinoma, high grade,* maxillary sinus. Closely packed glandular structures with hyperchromatic nuclei and focal necrosis

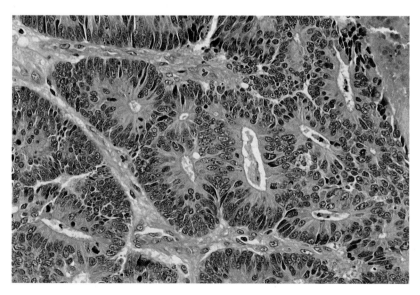

Fig. 58. *Adenocarcinoma, high grade,* maxillary sinus. Glandular structures with nuclear atypia and high mitotic activity. Same case as Fig. 57

130

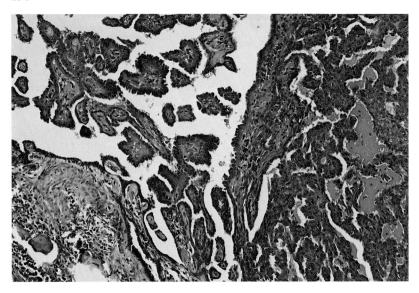

Fig. 59. *Papillary adenocarcinoma,* nasopharynx. Infiltrating papillary tumour occurring in continuity with nasopharyngeal surface epithelium

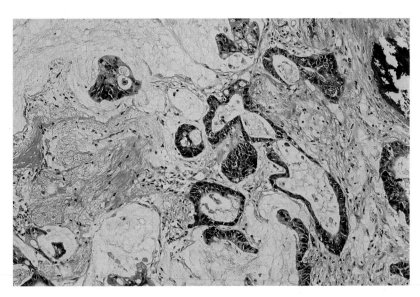

Fig. 60. *Mucinous adenocarcinoma,* ethmoid sinus. Poorly formed glandular structures in lakes of extracellular mucin

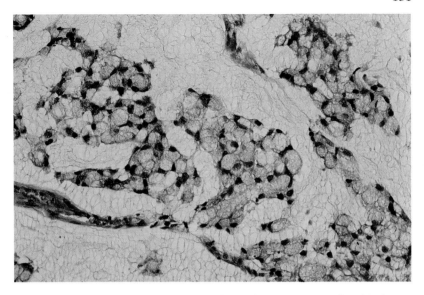

Fig. 61. *Mucinous adenocarcinoma,* maxillary sinus. Tumour cells with signet-ring morphology. Intracellular and extracellular mucin

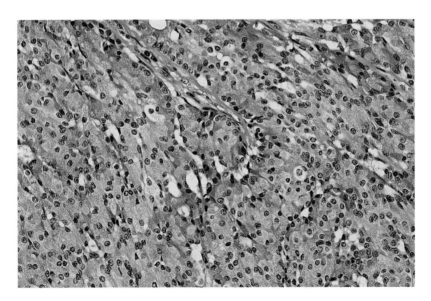

Fig. 62. *Acinic cell carcinoma,* nasal cavity. Mass of uniform polyhedral cells with basophilic granular cytoplasm. Fibrovascular stroma

132

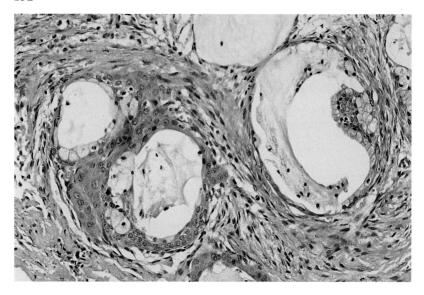

Fig. 63. *Mucoepidermoid carcinoma,* nasal cavity. Mucin-containing microcysts lined by squamous cells and mucous cells

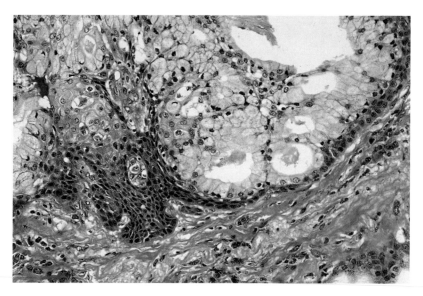

Fig. 64. *Mucoepidermoid carcinoma,* maxillary sinus. Tumour mass with admixture of squamous cells and mucous cells

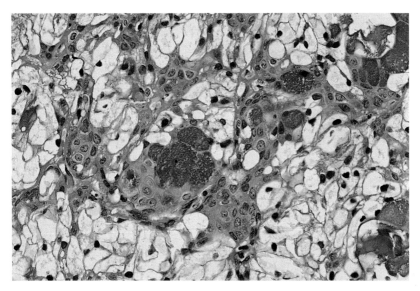

Fig. 65. *Mucoepidermoid carcinoma,* nasal cavity. Squamous cells, mucous cells and cells with clear cytoplasm. Mucicarmine

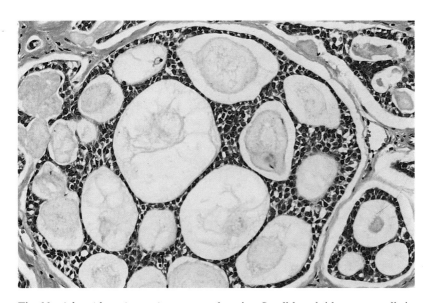

Fig. 66. *Adenoid cystic carcinoma,* nasal cavity. Small basaloid tumour cells in cribriform pattern

134

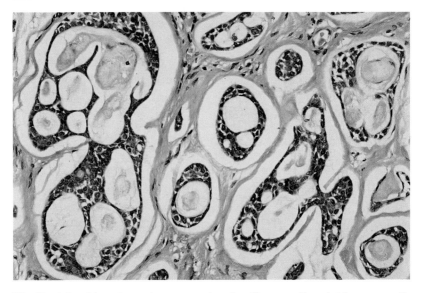

Fig. 67. *Adenoid cystic carcinoma,* nasal cavity. Groups of basaloid tumour cells in cribriform or cylindromatous pattern; sharply defined spaces containing mucohyaline material

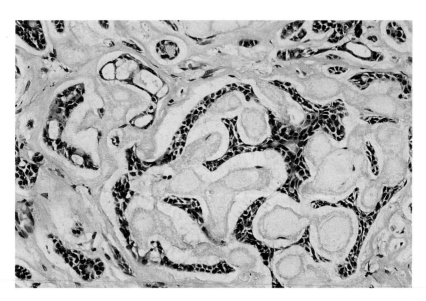

Fig. 68. *Adenoid cystic carcinoma,* nasal cavity. Trabecular structures separated by hyaline stroma

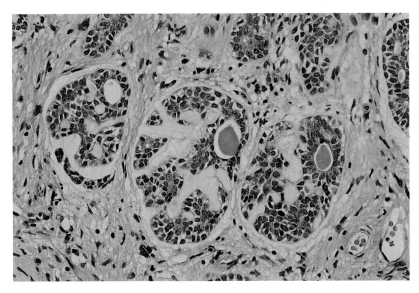

Fig. 69. *Adenoid cystic carcinoma,* maxillary sinus. Groups of tumour cells with sheaths of pale hyaline mucoid material and tubules containing mucin

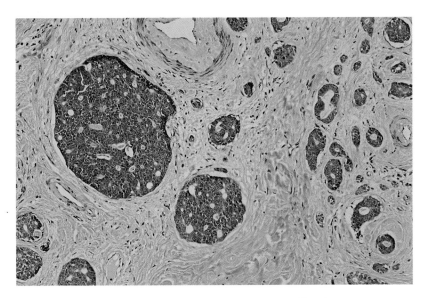

Fig. 70. *Adenoid cystic carcinoma,* maxillary sinus. Infiltrating tumour composed of uniform basaloid cells forming tubules and fenestrated compact masses

136

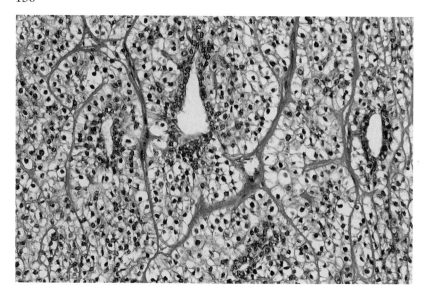

Fig. 71. *Epithelial-myoepithelial carcinoma,* nasal cavity. Epithelium-lined tubules surrounded by multilayered myoepithelial cells with abundant clear cytoplasm and sharply defined cell margins

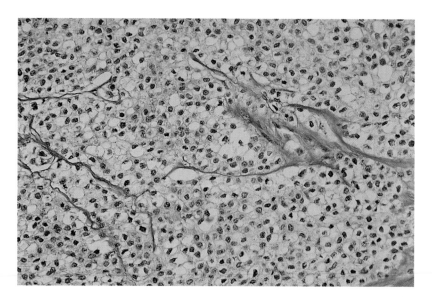

Fig. 72. *Clear cell carcinoma,* nasal cavity. Sheets of epithelial tumour cells with clear or vacuolated cytoplasm

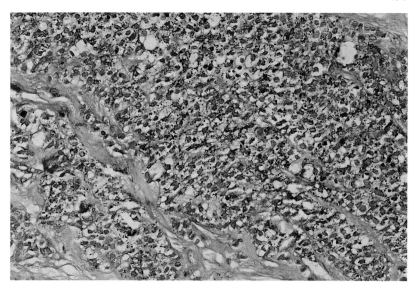

Fig. 73. *Clear cell carcinoma,* nasal cavity. Glycogen in tumour cells. Same case as Fig. 72. PAS

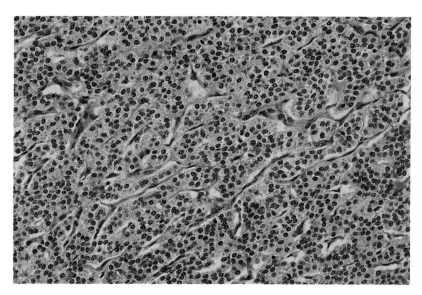

Fig. 74. *Carcinoid tumour,* trachea. Trabeculae of uniform cells with regular nuclei and granular cytoplasm. Vascular stroma

138

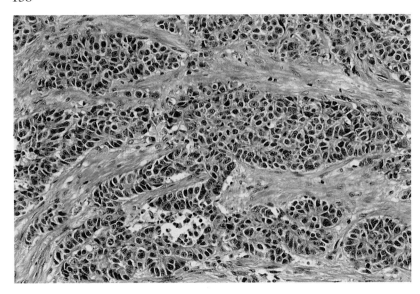

Fig. 75. *Atypical carcinoid tumour,* larynx. Infiltrating masses of moderately pleomorphic tumour cells with rosette-like structures and numerous mitoses

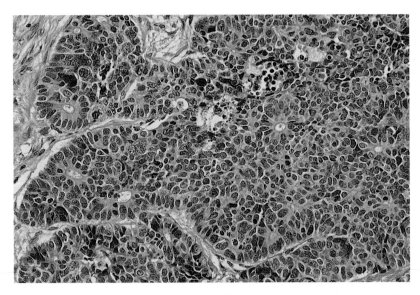

Fig. 76. *Atypical carcinoid tumour,* larynx. Tumour mass containing rosette-like glandular lumina and peripheral palisading. Pleomorphic tumour cells with hyperchromatic nuclei and numerous mitoses

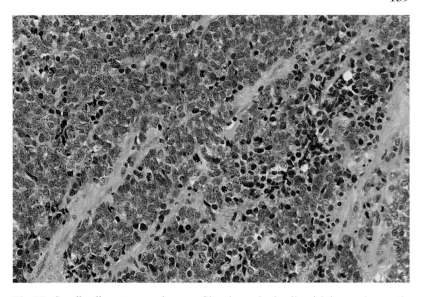

Fig. 77. *Small cell carcinoma,* larynx. Closely packed cells with hyperchromatic nuclei, inconspicuous nucleoli and scanty cytoplasm with poorly defined cell margins

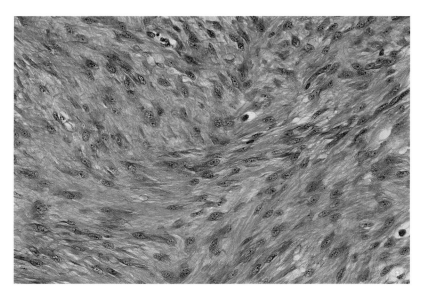

Fig. 78. *Aggressive fibromatosis.* Interwoven bundles of fibroblasts with bland cytologic features

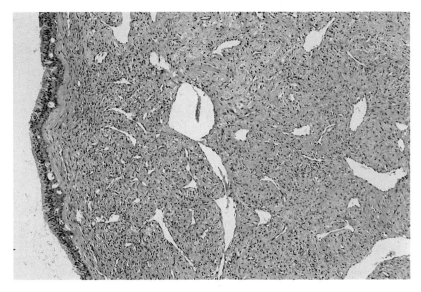

Fig. 79. *Angiofibroma,* posterolateral nasal wall. Tumour composed of capillary vessels of varying size and cellular fibrous tissue

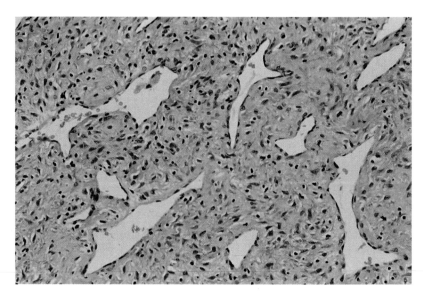

Fig. 80. *Angiofibroma,* posterolateral nasal wall. Gaping blood vessels devoid of muscle in cellular fibrous tissue. Same case as Fig. 79

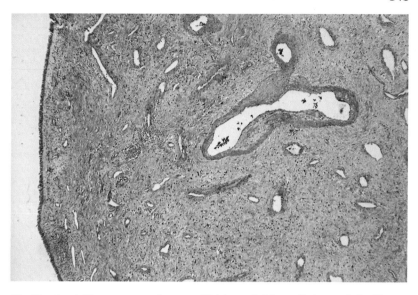

Fig. 81. *Angiofibroma,* nasopharynx. Thick- and thin-walled vessels in fibrous tissue. Focal intimal thickening

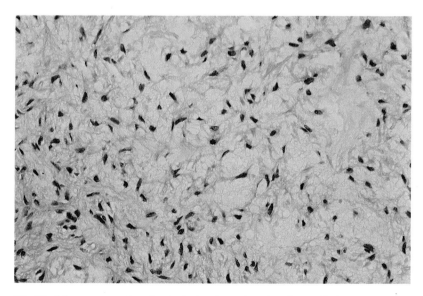

Fig. 82. *Myxoma,* nasal cavity. Spindle-shaped and stellate cells in an avascular myxoid matrix

142

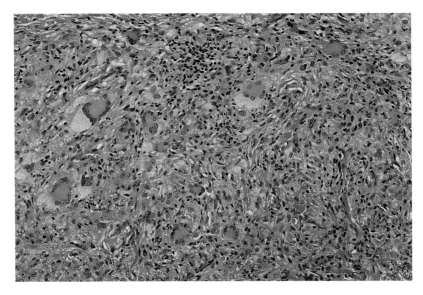

Fig. 83. *Fibrous histiocytoma,* nasal cavity. Tumour composed of fibroblasts, histiocytes and Touton-type giant cells with foamy cytoplasm. Focal lymphocytic infiltration

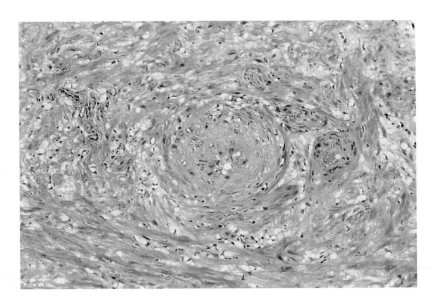

Fig. 84. *Vascular leiomyoma,* nasal cavity. Tumour composed of smooth muscle cells continuous with wall of blood vessel

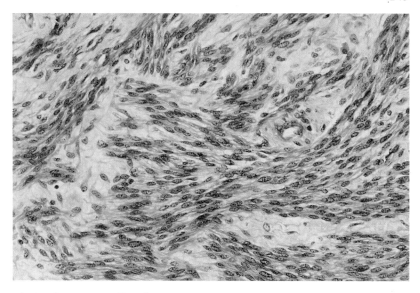

Fig. 85. *Leiomyoma.* Bundles of tumour cells with elongated blunt-ended nuclei and eosinophilic cytoplasm

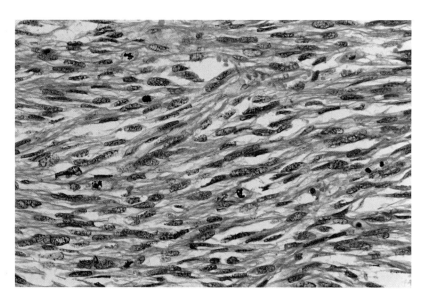

Fig. 86. *Leiomyosarcoma.* Spindle-shaped tumour cells with elongated blunt-ended nuclei, fibrillar eosinophilic cytoplasm and several mitoses

144

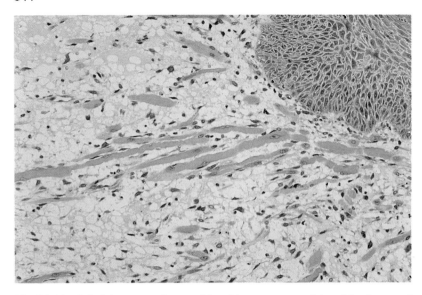

Fig. 87. *Fetal rhabdomyoma,* larynx. Myxoid tumour containing thin elongated muscle cells at periphery close to epithelial surface

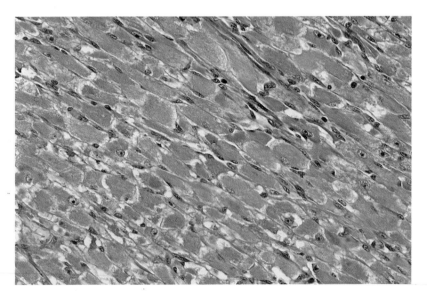

Fig. 88. *Adult rhabdomyoma,* larynx. Large muscle cells with abundant eosinophilic cytoplasm and vesicular peripherally placed nuclei. Glycogen vacuoles in some cells

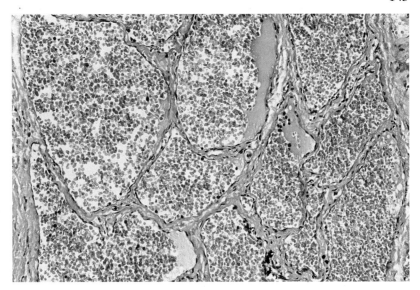

Fig. 89. *Haemangioma,* nasal cavity. Cavernous blood-filled endothelium-lined vessels

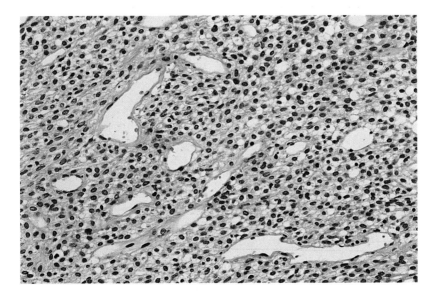

Fig. 90. *Haemangiopericytoma,* nasal cavity. Uniform tumour cells with regular nuclei and clear cytoplasm arranged around blood vessels lined by a single layer of endothelial cells

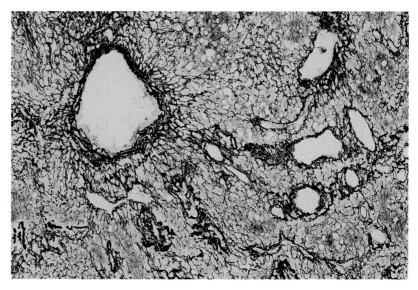

Fig. 91. *Haemangiopericytoma,* nasal cavity. Individual tumour cells and vascular basement membranes outlined by reticulin. Reticulin

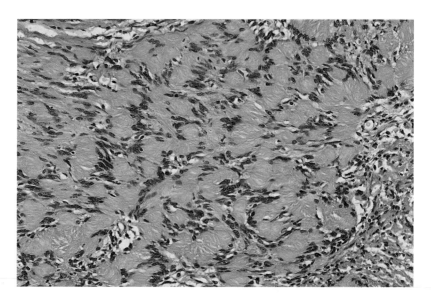

Fig. 92. *Neurilemmoma,* nasal cavity. Compact bundle of spindle-shaped tumour cells with nuclear palisading

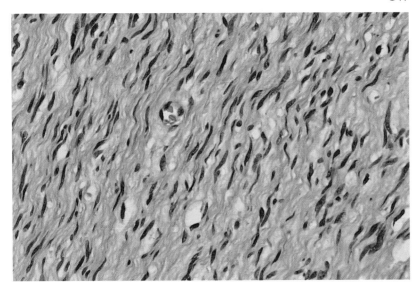

Fig. 93. *Neurofibroma,* nasopharynx. Bundle of spindle-shaped cells with elongated wavy or buckled nuclei with pointed ends

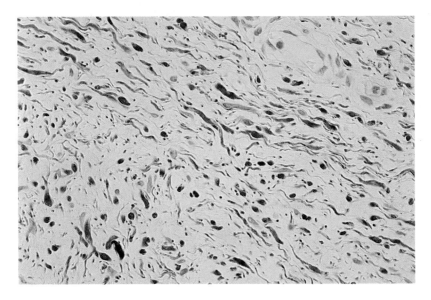

Fig. 94. *Neurofibroma,* nasopharynx. Tumour cells immunoreactive for S-100 protein. Same case as Fig. 93. Anti-S100

148

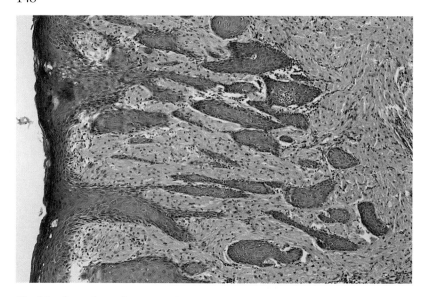

Fig. 95. *Granular cell tumour,* hypopharynx. Tumour cells with pale eosinophilic granular cytoplasm. Pseudoepitheliomatous hyperplasia of overlying stratified squamous epithelium

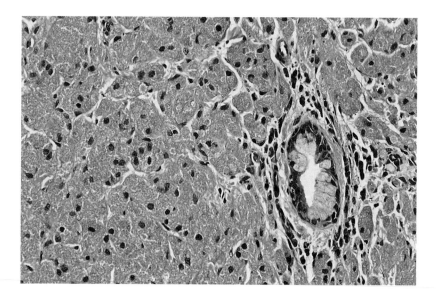

Fig. 96. *Granular cell tumour,* larynx. Tumour cells with pyknotic nuclei and abundant granular eosinophilic cytoplasm surrounding a laryngeal gland

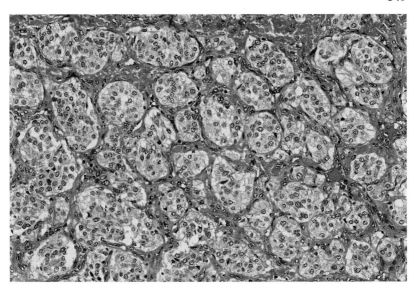

Fig. 97. *Paraganglioma,* middle ear. Nests of epithelioid tumour cells with finely granular pale cytoplasm separated by vascular stroma

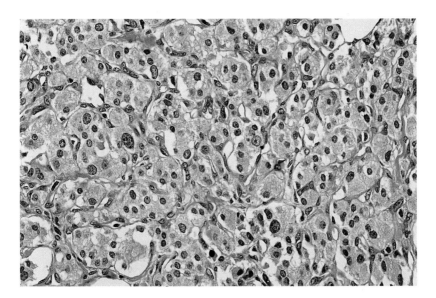

Fig. 98. *Paraganglioma,* nasopharynx. Irregular nests of cells with pleomorphic nuclei and pale granular cytoplasm separated by vascular stroma

150

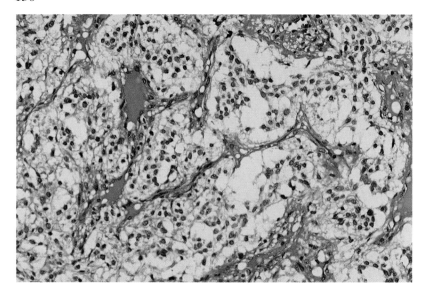

Fig. 99. *Paraganglioma,* middle ear. Tumour cells with abundant frayed cytoplasm with poorly defined cell margins

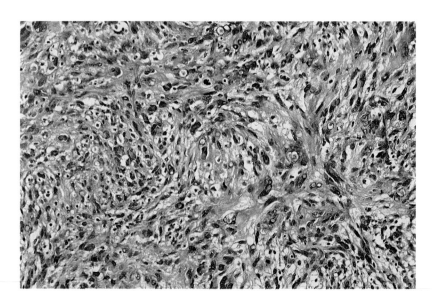

Fig. 100. *Malignant fibrous histiocytoma.* Pleomorphocellular sarcoma with storiform pattern

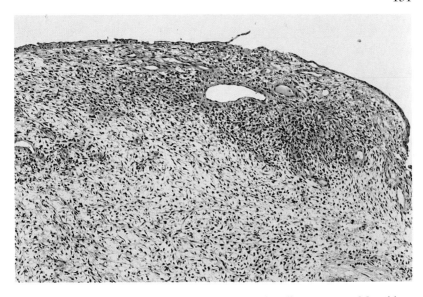

Fig. 101. *Embryonal rhabdomyosarcoma,* external auditory meatus. Myxoid tumour with a richly cellular zone close to epithelial surface

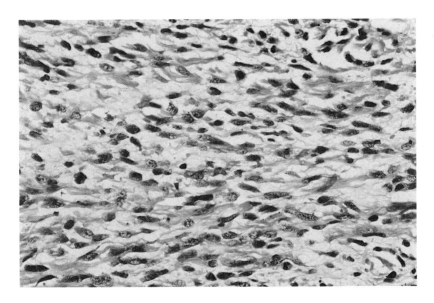

Fig. 102. *Embryonal rhabdomyosarcoma.* Loosely arranged spindle-shaped tumour cells with atypical hyperchromatic nuclei and eosinophilic cytoplasm

152

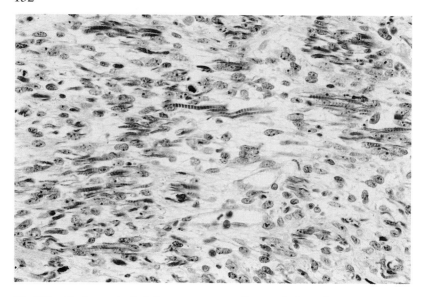

Fig. 103. *Embryonal rhabdomyosarcoma.* Cross-striations in tumour cells. Same case as Fig. 102. PTAH

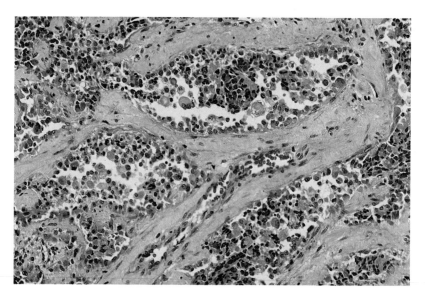

Fig. 104. *Alveolar rhabdomyosarcoma,* nasal cavity. Tumour cells arranged in well-defined alveolar masses separated by fibrous stroma. Centrally placed loose-lying tumour cells with eosinophilic cytoplasm

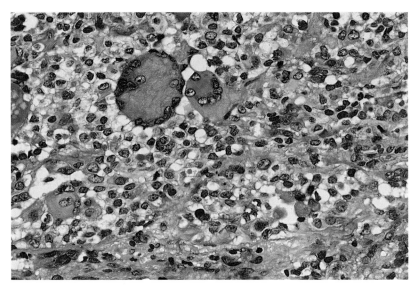

Fig. 105. *Alveolar rhabdomyosarcoma,* nasal cavity. Tumour cells with clear or vacuolated cytoplasm and tumour giant cells with peripherally placed nuclei

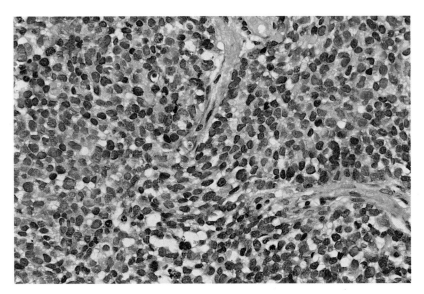

Fig. 106. *Alveolar rhabdomyosarcoma,* ethmoid sinus. Closely packed tumour cells with clear cytoplasm

154

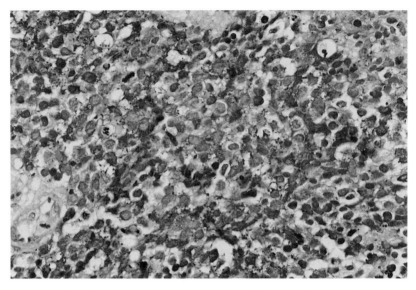

Fig. 107. *Alveolar rhabdomyosarcoma,* ethmoid sinus. Glycogen in tumour cells. Same case as Fig. 106. PAS

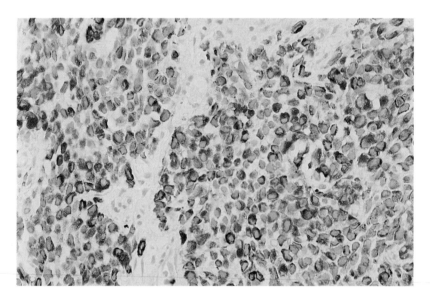

Fig. 108. *Alveolar rhabdomyosarcoma,* ethmoid sinus. Immunoreactive desmin in tumour cells. Anti-desmin

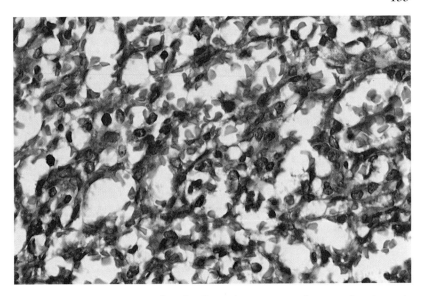

Fig. 109. *Angiosarcoma,* nasal cavity. Irregular anastomosing vascular channels lined by endothelial cells with atypical nuclei

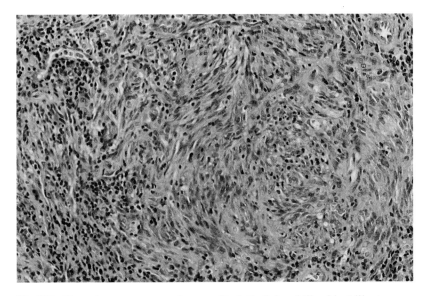

Fig. 110. *Kaposi sarcoma,* nasopharynx. Endothelial and fibroblast-like tumour cells with vascular slits. Extravasated red cells and lymphocytic infiltrates

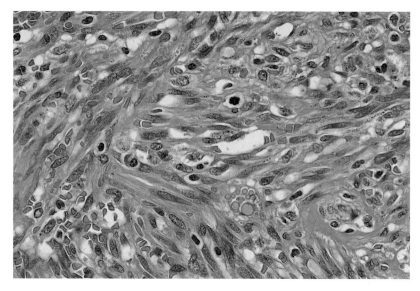

Fig. 111. *Kaposi sarcoma.* Spindle-shaped cells forming vascular slits. Hyaline globules and extravasated red cells

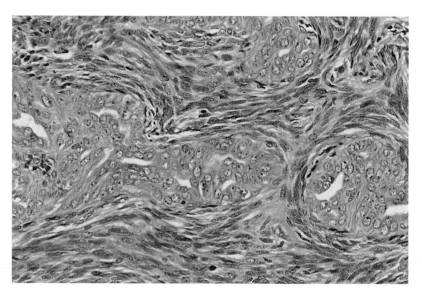

Fig. 112. *Synovial sarcoma,* hypopharynx. Epithelioid cells forming gland-like structures separated by a fibrosarcoma-like spindle cell component

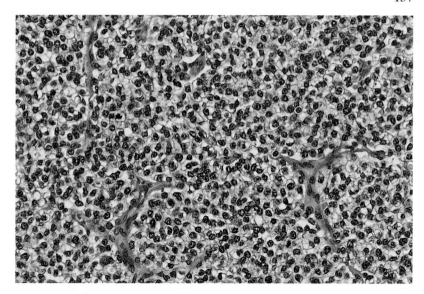

Fig. 113. *Ewing sarcoma.* Mass of closely packed uniform small cells with vacuolated cytoplasm

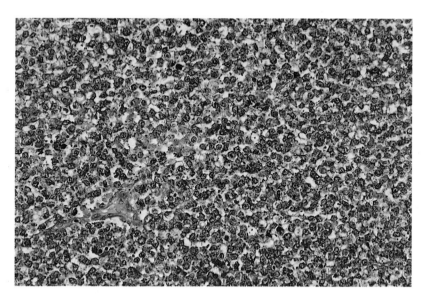

Fig. 114. *Ewing sarcoma.* Glycogen in tumour cells. Same case as Fig. 113. PAS

158

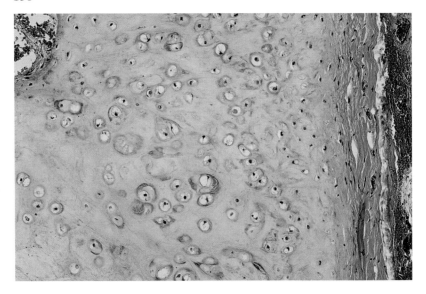

Fig. 115. *Chondroma,* larynx. Well-defined mass of mature cartilage

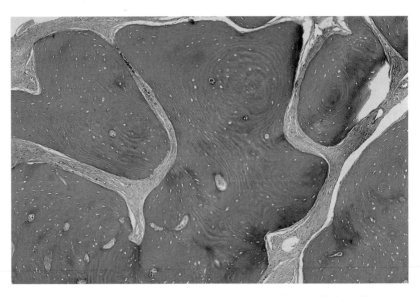

Fig. 116. *Osteoma,* external auditory meatus. Mature bone with lamellar structure

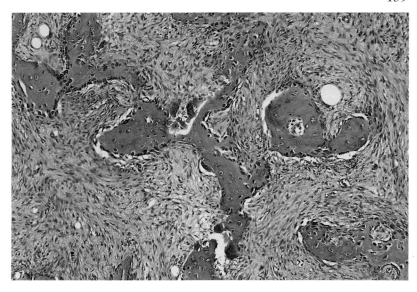

Fig. 117. *Ossifying fibroma,* maxilla. Cellular fibrous tissue containing trabeculae of bone rimmed by osteoblasts

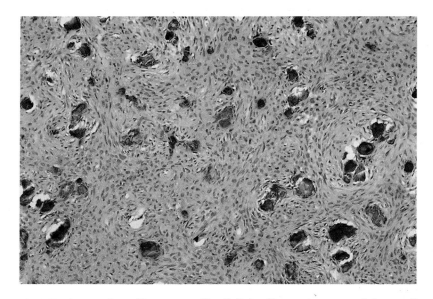

Fig. 118. *Cementifying fibroma,* maxilla. Cellular fibrous tissue containing small heavily mineralized cementum-like masses

160

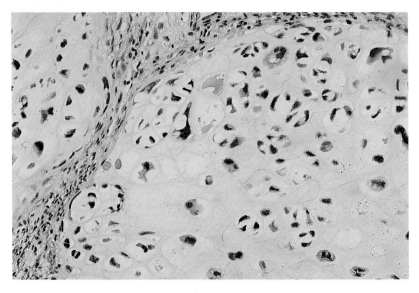

Fig. 119. *Chondrosarcoma,* larynx. Cartilaginous tumour with nuclear atypia, pleomorphism and mitotic activity

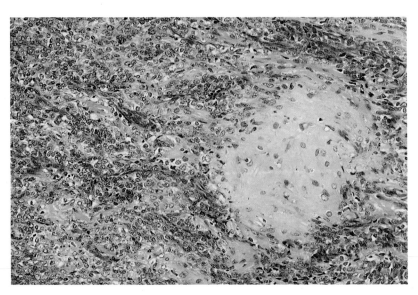

Fig. 120. *Mesenchymal chondrosarcoma.* Island of chondroid tissue in a highly vascular tumour composed of undifferentiated mesenchymal cells

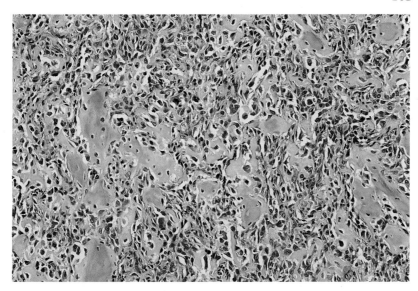

Fig. 121. *Osteosarcoma,* maxilla. Pleomorphocellular sarcoma with osteoid formation by tumour cells

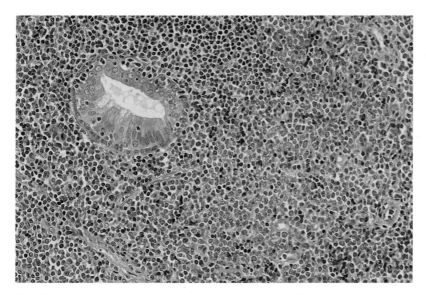

Fig. 122. *Malignant lymphoma, mixed small and large cell (centroblastic-centrocytic), diffuse,* nasopharynx. Tumour comprising small lymphocytes, cleaved cells and blasts. Invasion of glandular epithelium

162

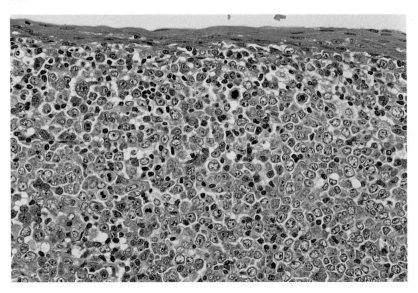

Fig. 123. *Malignant lymphoma, large cell (centroblastic), diffuse,* nasal cavity. Large lymphoid cells with pale staining nuclei

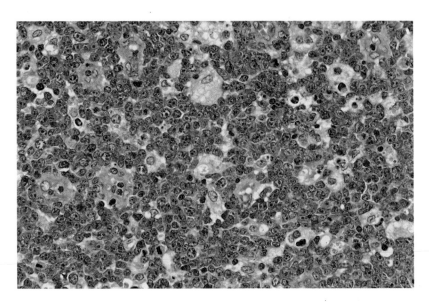

Fig. 124. *Malignant lymphoma, small non-cleaved cell (B-lymphoblastic), Burkitt-type,* maxilla. Sheet of lymphoblasts with a starry-sky pattern due to presence of scattered foamy macrophages

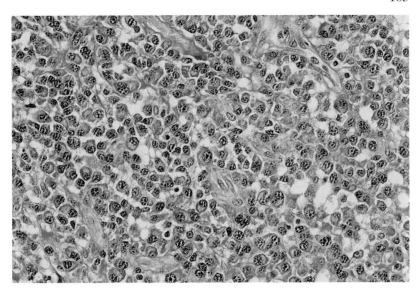

Fig. 125. *Extramedullary plasmacytoma,* nasopharynx. Tumour composed exclusively of fairly mature plasma cells

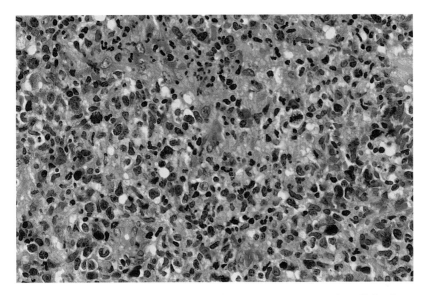

Fig. 126. *Midline malignant reticulosis,* nasal cavity. Pleomorphocellular lymphoma with infiltration by inflammatory cells

164

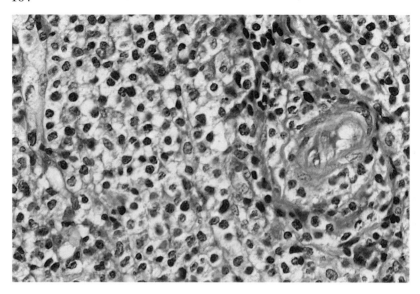

Fig. 127. *Midline malignant reticulosis,* nasal cavity. Lymphoma cells occurring in sheets and forming a cuff around a blood vessel

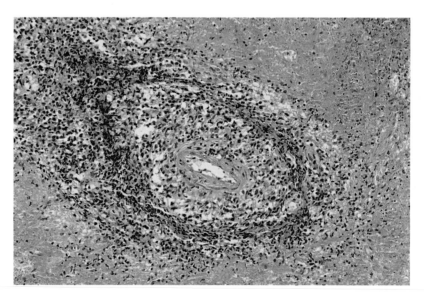

Fig. 128. *Midline malignant reticulosis,* nasal cavity. Angioinvasive lymphoma with necrosis

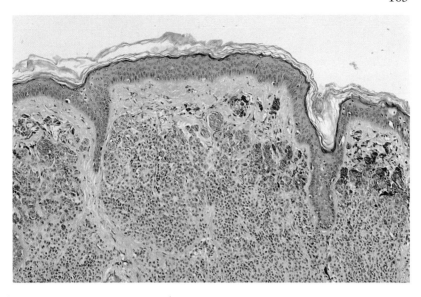

Fig. 129. *Melanocytic naevus,* pinna. Aggregates of naevus cells, some heavily pigmented, in dermis

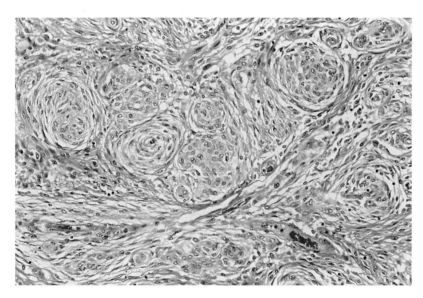

Fig. 130. *Meningioma,* nasal cavity. Nests and perivascular whorls of meningo-thelial cells

166

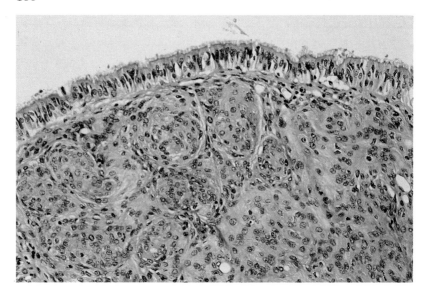

Fig. 131. *Meningioma,* nasal cavity. Nests of meningothelial cells in nasal mucosa

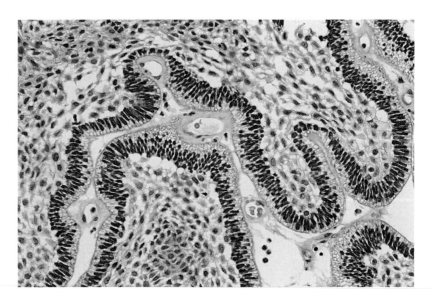

Fig. 132. *Ameloblastoma,* maxillary sinus. Loosely packed stellate cells surrounded by a palisaded layer of columnar cells

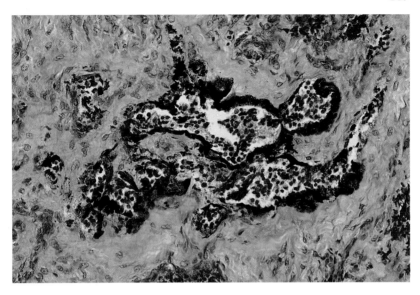

Fig. 133. *Melanotic neuroectodermal tumour,* maxilla. Small neuroblast-like cells within irregular alveolar spaces lined by heavily pigmented cells. Fibrous stroma

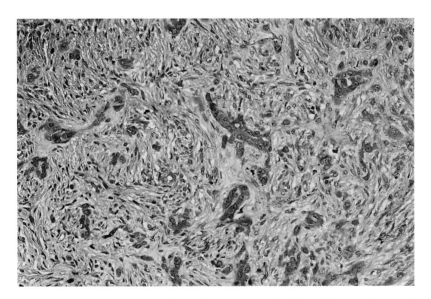

Fig. 134. *Melanotic neuroectodermal tumour,* maxilla. Duct-like structures and cords of cuboidal cells separated by fibrous stroma

168

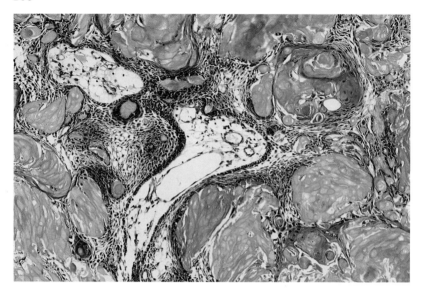

Fig. 135. *Craniopharyngioma,* nasopharynx. Masses of keratin within tumour masses composed of loosely packed stellate epithelial cells surrounded by a palisaded basal layer bordering an oedematous stroma

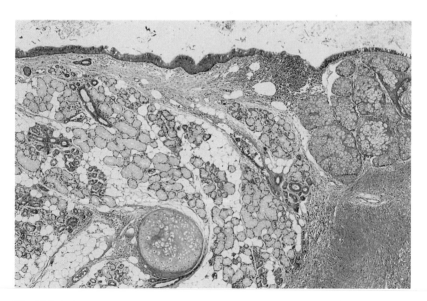

Fig. 136. *Mature teratoma,* nasal cavity. Tumour containing mature glial tissue, cartilage, fat, seromucinous glands, sebaceous glands and a cyst lined by pseudostratified ciliated epithelium

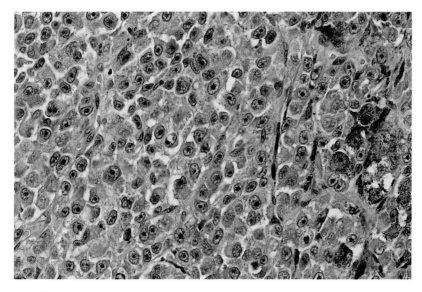

Fig. 137. *Malignant melanoma,* nasal cavity. Pigmented and non-pigmented tumour cells with vesicular nuclei and prominent nucleoli

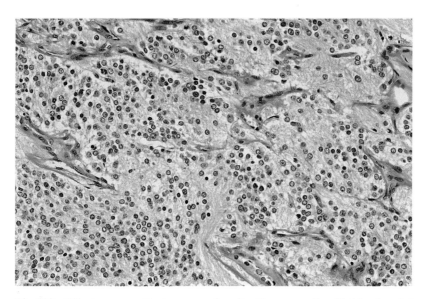

Fig. 138. *Olfactory neuroblastoma,* nasal cavity. Tumour cells with bland nuclei and abundant neurofibrils

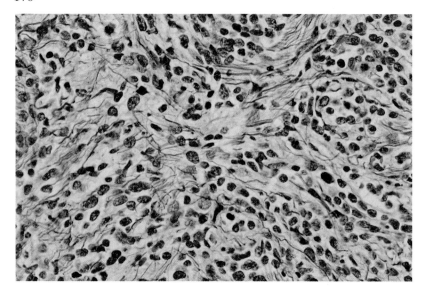

Fig. 139. *Olfactory neuroblastoma,* nasal cavity. Neurofibrils among tumour cells. Bodian

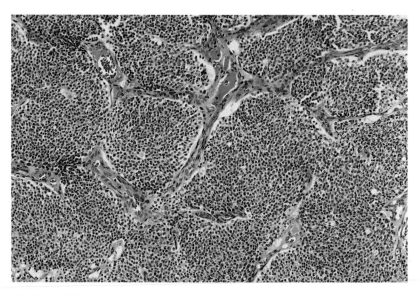

Fig. 140. *Olfactory neuroblastoma,* nasal cavity. Lobulated masses of closely packed small cells separated by fibrous stroma

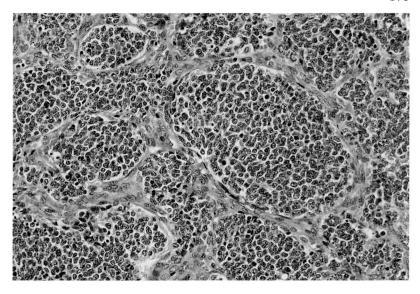

Fig. 141. *Olfactory neuroblastoma,* nasal cavity. Poorly differentiated neuroblasts without neurofibrils. Numerous mitoses. Lobular pattern with vascular stroma

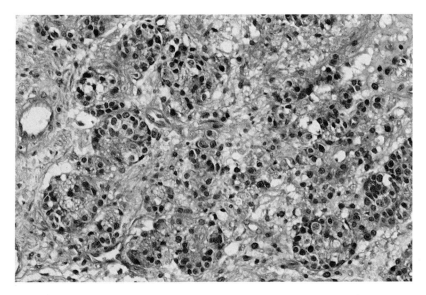

Fig. 142. *Olfactory neuroblastoma,* nasal cavity. Neuroblasts forming Homer Wright rosettes with central fibrillary material

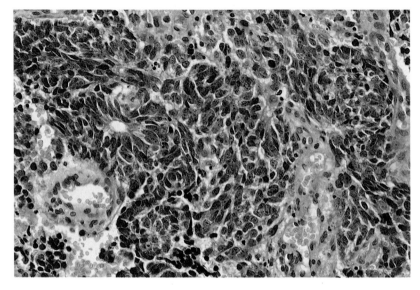

Fig.143. *Olfactory neuroblastoma,* nasal cavity. Poorly differentiated neuro-blasts forming Flexner-type rosette with central lumen

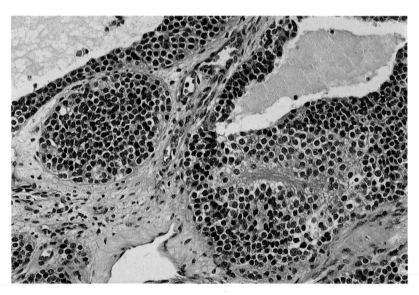

Fig.144. *Olfactory neuroblastoma,* nasal cavity. Lobular masses of neuroblasts and neurofibrils containing pseudocystic spaces

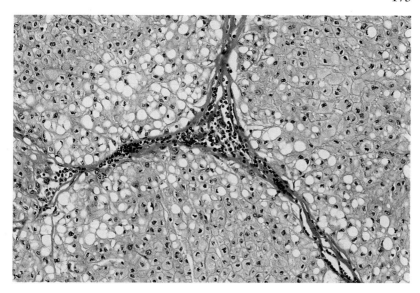

Fig. 145. *Chordoma,* nasopharynx. Lobular masses of closely packed polyhedral cells with abundant occasionally vacuolated cytoplasm and well-defined cell margins

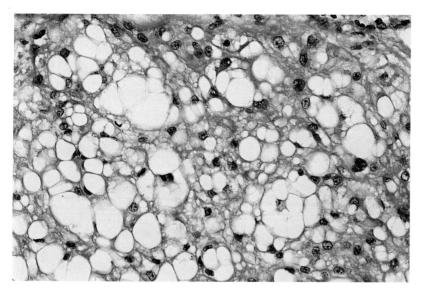

Fig. 146. *Chordoma,* nasopharynx. Large cells with markedly vacuolated bubbly cytoplasm

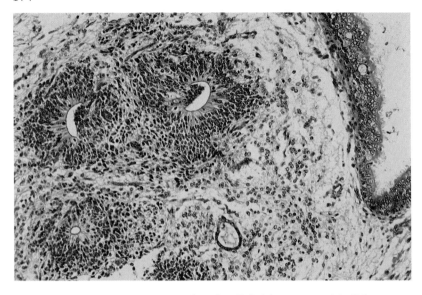

Fig. 147. *Immature teratoma,* nasal cavity. Primitive neuroepithelial rosettes lined by multilayered neuroblasts with high mitotic activity. Part of cyst lined by ciliated pseudostratified epithelium

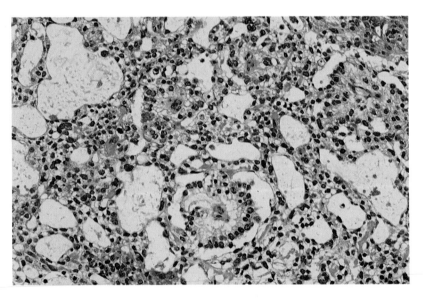

Fig. 148. *Yolk sac tumour.* Primitive vacuolated cells forming microcysts and a Schiller-Duval body. Intracellular and extracellular eosinophilic hyaline globules

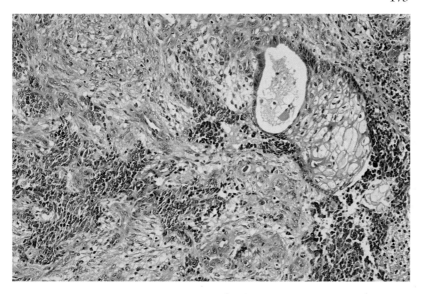

Fig. 149. *Teratocarcinosarcoma,* ethmoid sinus. Epithelial structure formed by vacuolated squamous cells and columnar cells, infiltrates of immature mesen-chymal cells and fibrovascular stroma

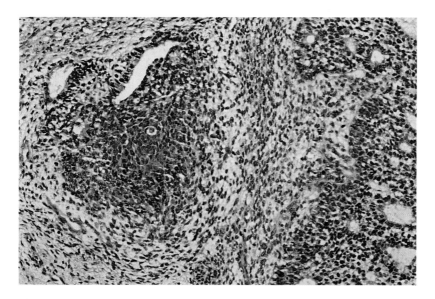

Fig. 150. *Teratocarcinosarcoma,* ethmoid sinus. Glandular structures lined by cuboidal and columnar epithelium and sarcoma-like areas resembling primitive mesenchyme

176

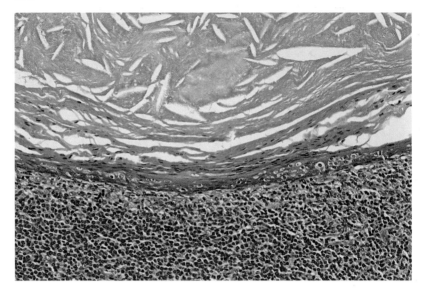

Fig. 151. *Branchial cleft cyst,* nasopharynx. Cyst lined by keratinizing stratified squamous epithelium. Lymphoid tissue in cyst wall

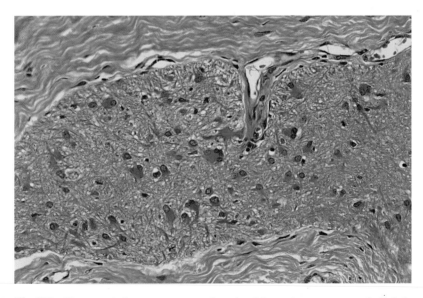

Fig. 152. *Heterotopic brain tissue,* nasal cavity. Mass of astrocytes and glial fibres

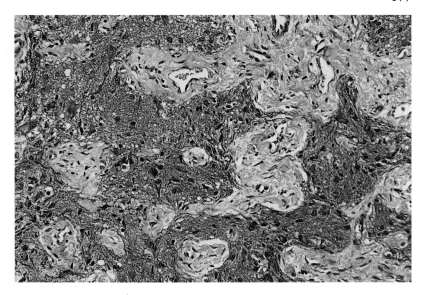

Fig. 153. *Heterotopic brain tissue,* nasal cavity. Bands of astrocytes and glial fibres in fibrous stroma. PTAH

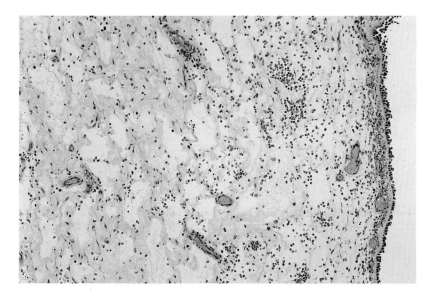

Fig. 154. *Inflammatory sinonasal polyp.* Oedematous mucosa infiltrated by eosinophil leucocytes

178

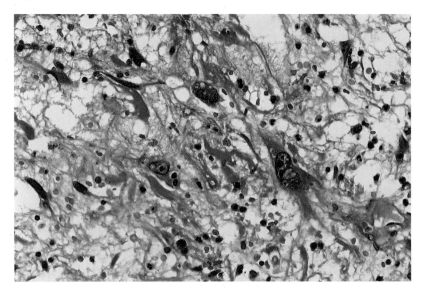

Fig. 155. *Inflammatory sinonasal polyp.* Atypical fibroblasts with bizarre nuclei

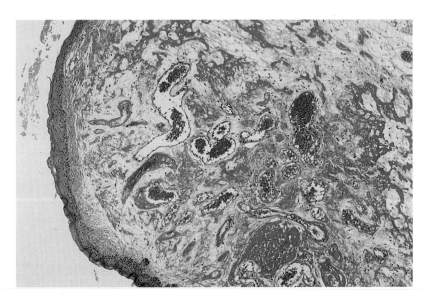

Fig. 156. *Vocal cord polyp.* Polyp containing dilated blood vessels and stromal deposits of eosinophilic hyaline material

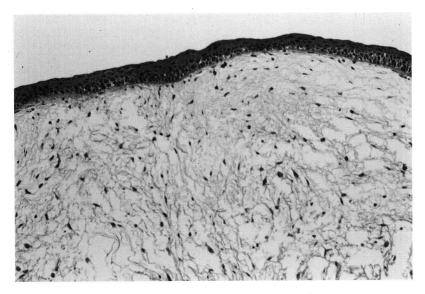

Fig. 157. *Vocal cord polyp.* Polyp with myxoid structure

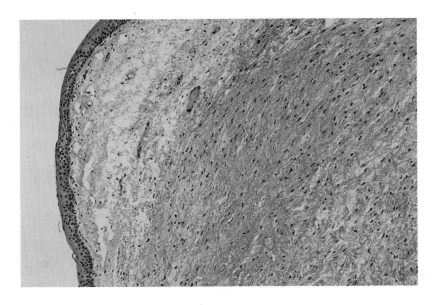

Fig. 158. *Vocal cord polyp.* Polyp with fibrous structure

180

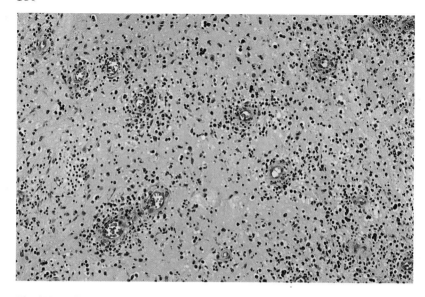

Fig. 159. *Inflammatory otic polyp.* Oedematous granulation tissue with infiltration by inflammatory cells

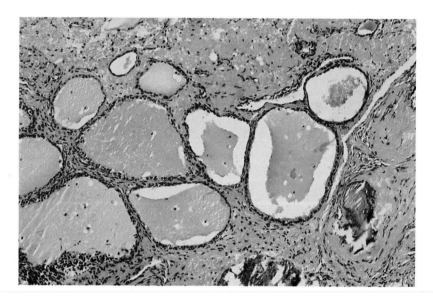

Fig. 160. *Inflammatory otic polyp.* Metaplastic gland-like structures found at base of inflammatory otic polyp

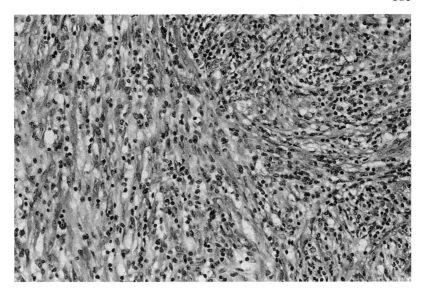

Fig. 161. *Fibro-inflammatory pseudotumour,* maxillary sinus. Fibroblasts with heavy infiltration by lymphocytes and plasma cells

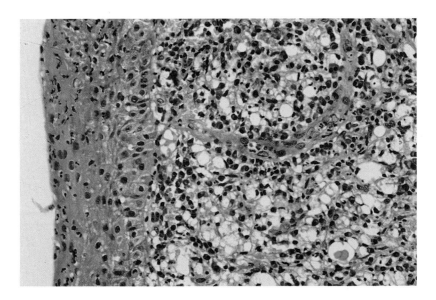

Fig. 162. *Scleroma,* nasal mucosa. Large vacuolated macrophages (Mikulicz cells) and plasma cells

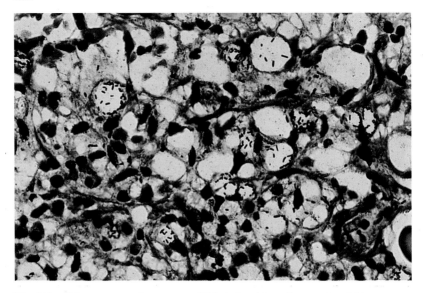

Fig. 163. *Scleroma*, nasal mucosa. *Klebsiella rhinoscleromatis* within macrophages. Warthin-Starry

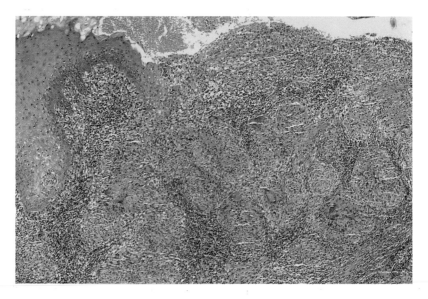

Fig. 164. *Tuberculosis*, larynx. Granulomas with Langhans giant cells at base of laryngeal ulcer

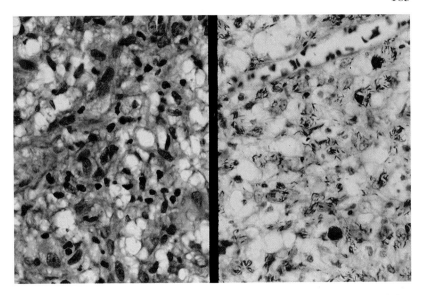

Fig. 165. *Lepromatous leprosy*, nasal mucosa. Foamy macrophages containing numerous acid-fast bacilli. H & E/Fite-Faraco

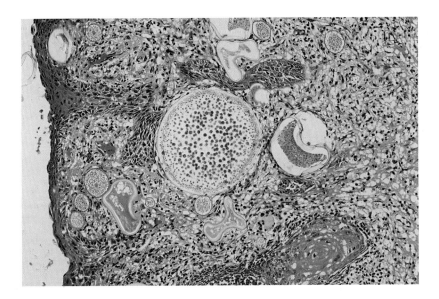

Fig. 166. *Rhinosporidiosis*, nasal mucosa. Sporangia in various stages of development containing spores of *Rhinosporidium seeberi*

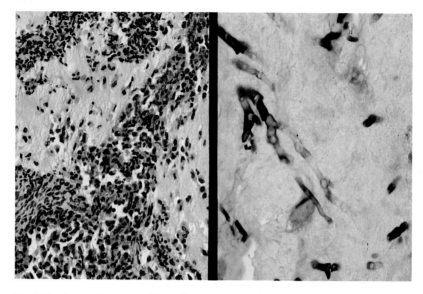

Fig. 167. *Aspergillosis,* maxillary sinus. Inspissated mucus containing eosinophil leucocytes, necrotic cells and aspergillus hyphae. H & E × 250/Gomori × 600

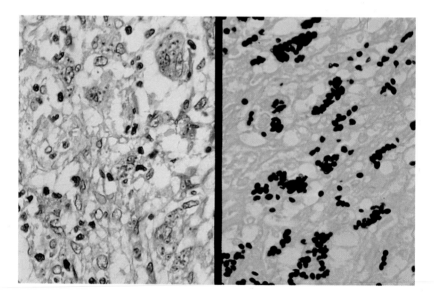

Fig. 168. *Histoplasmosis,* larynx. Macrophages containing Histoplasma capsulatum. PAS/Gomori

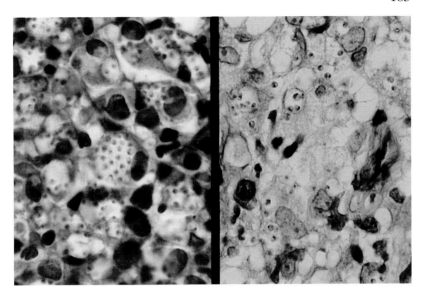

Fig. 169. *Leishmaniasis,* nasal mucosa. Macrophages containing *Leishmania braziliensis.* H & E/Giemsa

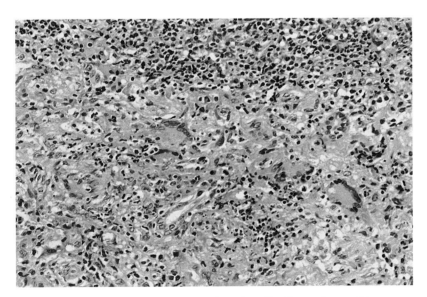

Fig. 170. *Wegener granulomatosis,* nasal mucosa. Small vessel vasculitis, granu-lomas containing Langhans-type giant cells and infiltration by inflammatory cells

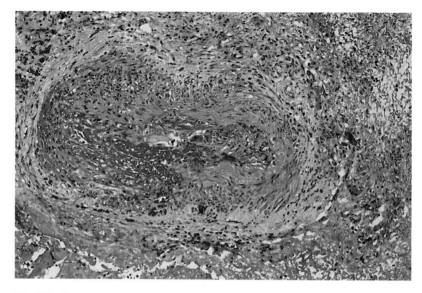

Fig. 171. *Wegener granulomatosis,* nasal mucosa. Vasculitis and fibrinoid necrosis in artery adjoining necrotic area

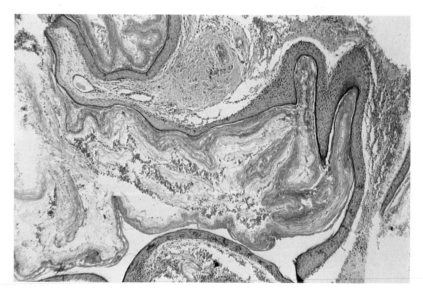

Fig. 172. *Epidermoid cholesteatoma,* middle ear. Laminated mass of keratin in cavity lined by squamous epithelium

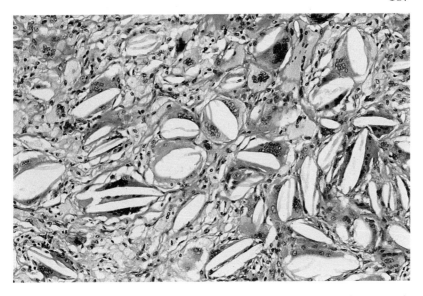

Fig. 173. *Cholesterol granuloma,* middle ear. Foreign body giant cells surrounding cholesterol clefts

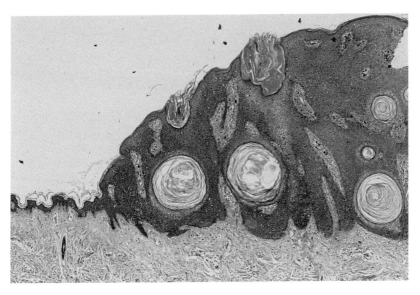

Fig. 174. *Seborrhoeic keratosis,* pinna. Skin lesion projecting above level of epidermis and consisting of basaloid cells and sharply defined keratin cysts

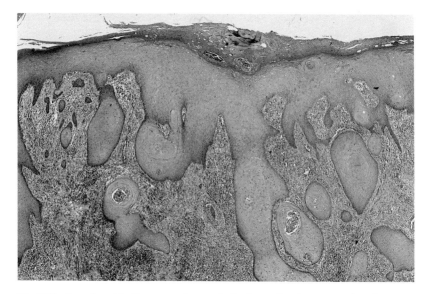

Fig. 175. *Pseudoepitheliomatous hyperplasia.* Irregular downgrowths of mature squamous epithelium in case of chromomycosis

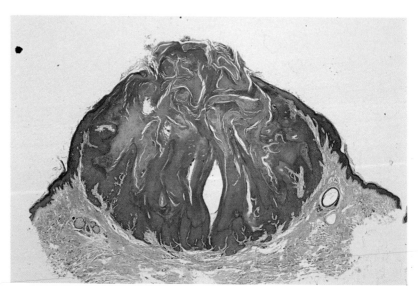

Fig. 176. *Keratoacanthoma,* pinna. Raised skin lesion with cup-shaped downgrowth of squamous epithelium into dermis. Central keratin-filled crater with overhanging lips of epidermis

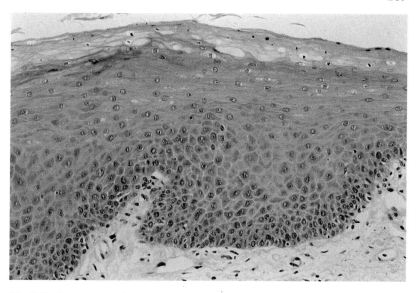

Fig. 177. *Squamous cell hyperplasia,* larynx. Increase in cell layers of squamous epithelium with normal maturation. Keratosis

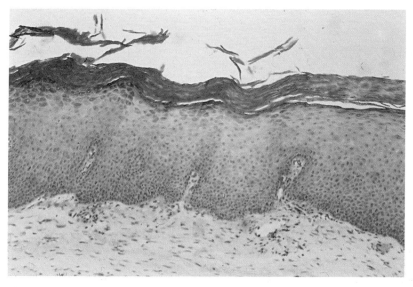

Fig. 178. *Keratosis,* larynx. Thick layer of keratin over squamous epithelium. Increase in cell layers with normal maturation

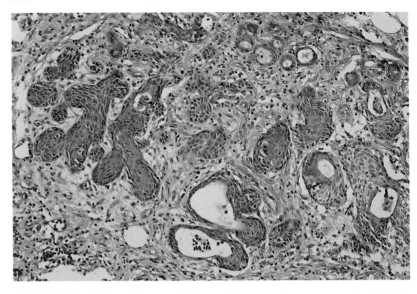

Fig. 179. *Necrotizing sialometaplasia,* nasal mucosa. Squamous metaplasia involving ducts and acini of seromucinous gland

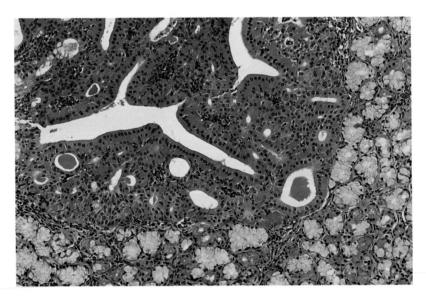

Fig. 180. *Oncocytic hyperplasia,* nasopharynx. Seromucinous gland partly replaced by glandular units composed of cells with abundant eosinophilic cytoplasm

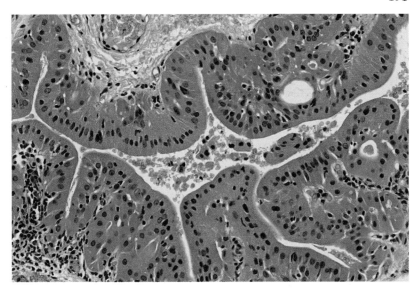

Fig. 181. *"Oncocytic papillary cystadenoma"*, larynx. Laryngeal cyst lined by bi-layered oncocytic epithelium

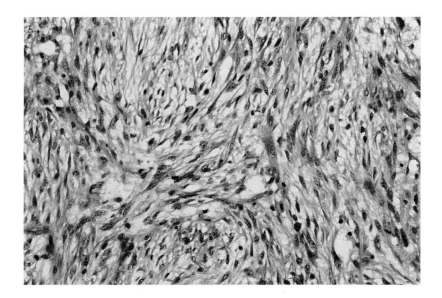

Fig. 182. *Nodular fasciitis,* nasal cavity. Loosely arranged waves of proliferating fibroblasts

192

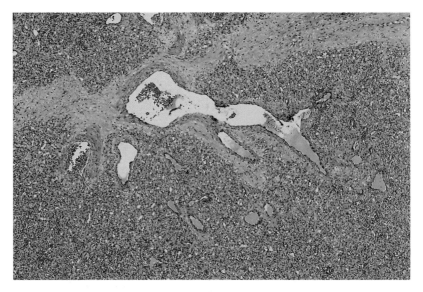

Fig. 183. *Granuloma pyogenicum,* nasal mucosa. Lobules of capillaries with feeder vessels

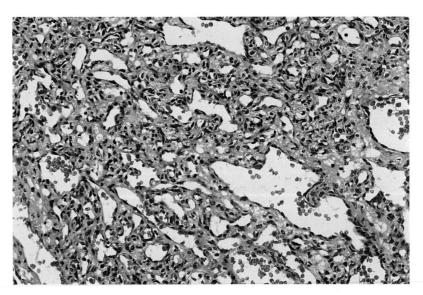

Fig. 184. *Granuloma pyogenicum,* nasal mucosa. Closely packed capillaries with inflammatory cells in stroma

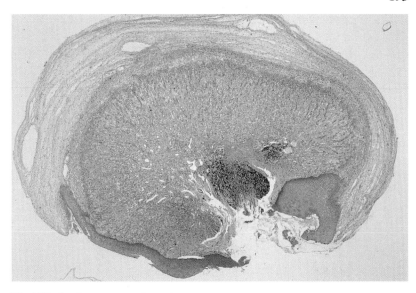

Fig. 185. *Intubation granuloma,* larynx. Fibrin-covered polypoid mass of granulation tissue overlying laryngeal ulcer. Aggregates of haemosiderin pigment at base

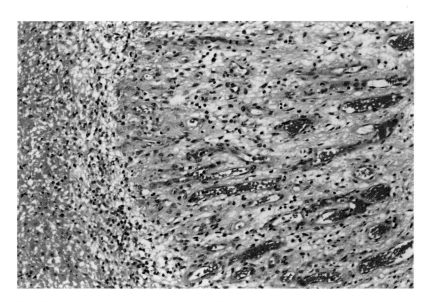

Fig. 186. *Intubation granuloma,* larynx. Vascular granulation tissue covered by necrotic inflammatory exudate

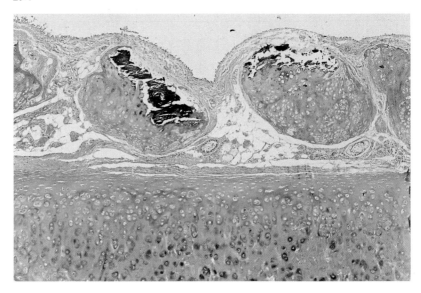

Fig. 187. *Tracheopathia osteochondroplastica.* Submucous nodules of calcifying cartilage

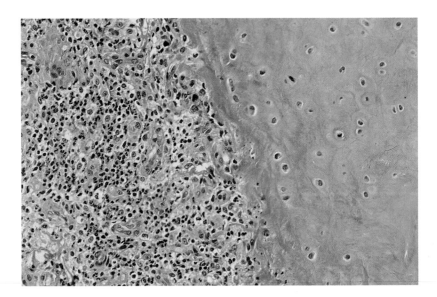

Fig. 188. *Chondrodermatitis nodularis helicis.* Perichondrial inflammation

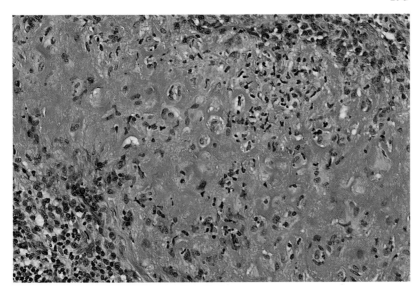

Fig. 189. *Relapsing polychondritis,* auricular cartilage. Degenerative changes in cartilage associated with inflammatory infiltrate comprising plasma cells and lymphocytes

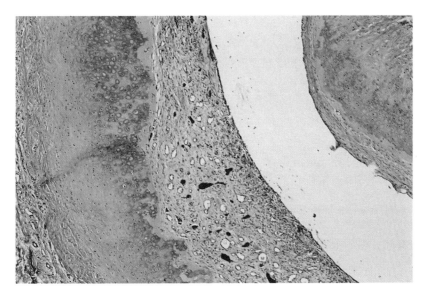

Fig. 190. *Cystic chondromalacia,* auricular cartilage. Granulation tissue-lined pseudocyst within cartilage

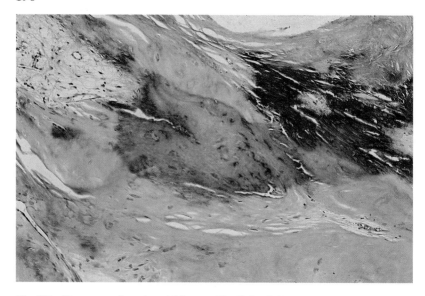

Fig. 191. *Tympanosclerosis,* middle ear. Hyalinized fibrous tissue with calcification

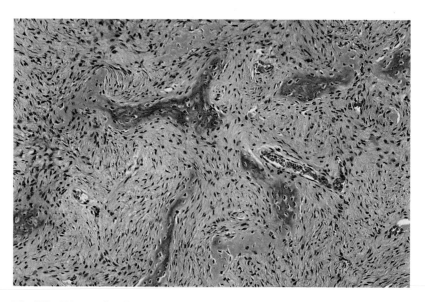

Fig. 192. *Fibrous dysplasia,* maxilla. Cellular fibrous tissue containing irregular trabeculae of metaplastic woven bone

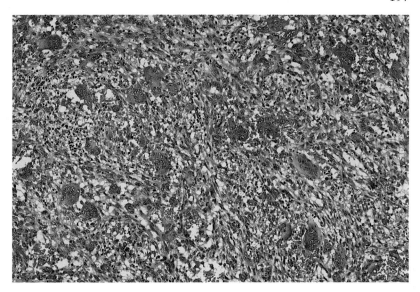

Fig. 193. *Giant cell reparative granuloma,* maxilla. Cellular fibrous tissue containing aggregates of multinucleated osteoclast-like giant cells

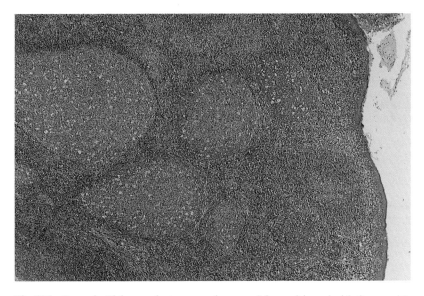

Fig. 194. *Lymphoid hyperplasia,* nasopharynx. Mass of lymphoid tissue with germinal centres

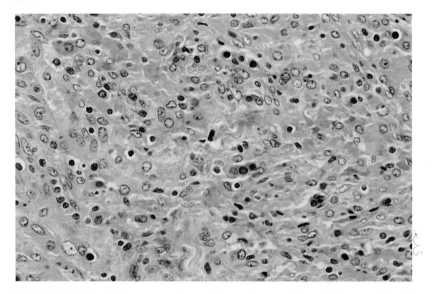

Fig. 195. *Malakoplakia,* external ear. Macrophages with vesicular nuclei and eosinophilic cytoplasm. Numerous deeply staining intracellular and extracellular rounded concretions (Michaelis-Gutmann bodies)

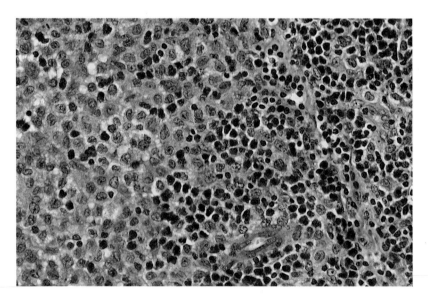

Fig. 196. *Langerhans cell histiocytosis,* middle ear. Meshwork of histiocytes with pale grooved nuclei. Aggregates of eosinophils and lymphocytes

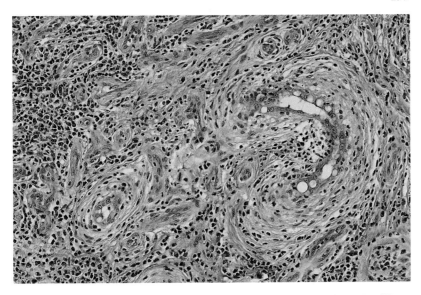

Fig. 197. *Angiolymphoid hyperplasia with eosinophilia,* external ear. Proliferation of vessels lined by endothelial cells with epithelioid features. Infiltrates of eosinophils and lymphocytes

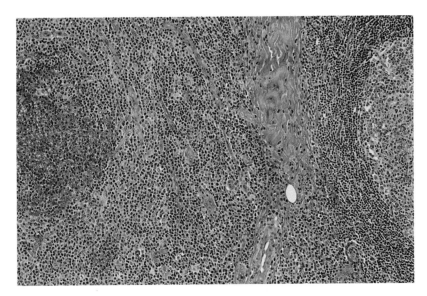

Fig. 198. *Kimura disease,* external ear. Lymphocytic infiltrates with formation of germinal centres. Heavy infiltration by eosinophils and eosinophilic folliculo-lysis

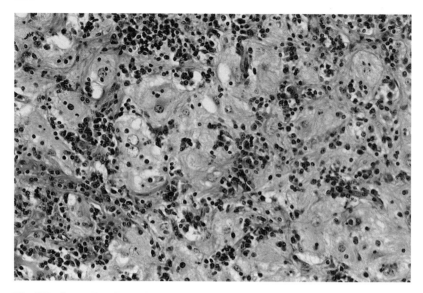

Fig. 199. *Rosai-Dorfman disease,* nasal cavity. Histiocytes with vesicular nuclei and abundant foamy cytoplasm containing lymphocytes. Numerous plasma cells

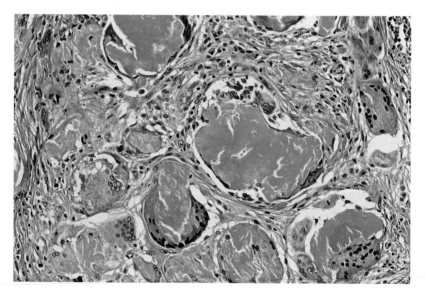

Fig. 200. *Amyloid deposit,* nasopharynx. Hyaline eosinophilic masses of amyloid with foreign body giant cells

WHO International Histological Classification of Tumours
Shanmugaratnam et al.: Histological Typing of Tumours
of the Upper Respiratory Tract and Ear, 2nd ed.

---

35 mm Colour Transparencies

A set of 200 colour slides (35 mm), corresponding to the photo-micrographs in this book, is available from the American Registry of Pathology. To order these *slides,* send the following information to:

American Registry of Pathology
14th Street and Alaska Ave. NW
Washington, DC 20306 USA

Please send me:

_____ set(s) of 35 mm slides of Histological Typing of Tumours of the Upper Respiratory Tract and Ear at $ 125 per set.
For Air Mail outside of North America add $ 10.

Total cost: $ _____ .00

Name _____

Address _____

_____

_____

Date _____ Signature _____

☐ I enclose a check/money order in US$ payable to the ARP.
☐ Please charge my credit card:
  ☐ VISA
  ☐ MasterCard

Card number _____

Expiration date _____

Name as it appears on credit card _____

Prices are subject to change without notice.

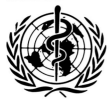

World Health Organization
International Histological
Classification of Tumours

Histological Typing of . . .

C. Hedinger
Histological Typing of
Thyroid Tumours
In Collaboration with E. D. Williams
and L. H. Sobin
2nd ed. 1988. XII, 67 pp. 92 figs. Softcover.
ISBN 3-540-19244-1

J. R. Jass, L. H. Sobin
Histological Typing of
Intestinal Tumours
2nd ed. 1989. XII, 127 pp. 136 figs. Softcover.
ISBN 3-540-50711-6

H. Watanabe, J. R. Jass, L. H. Sobin
Histological Typing of
Oesophageal and
Gastric Tumours
2nd ed. 1990. XII, 109 pp. 120 figs. 4 tabs.
Softcover. ISBN 3-540-51629-8

J. Albores-Saavedra, D. E. Henson, L. H. Sobin
Histological Typing of
Tumours of the
Gallbladder and
Extrahepatic Bile Ducts
2nd ed. 1991. XI, 77 pp. 80 figs. Softcover.
ISBN 3-540-52838-5

K. Shanmugaratnam
Histological Typing of
Tumours of the Upper
Respiratory Tract and Ear
In Collaboration with L. H. Sobin
2nd ed. 1991. Approx. 160 pp. 200 figs.
Softcover. ISBN 3-540-53880-1

G. Seifert
Histological Typing of
Salivary Gland Tumours
In Collaboration with L. H. Sobin
2nd ed. 1991. XI, 112 pp. 130 figs. Softcover.
ISBN 3-540-54031-8

I. R. H. Kramer, J. J. Pindborg, M. Shear
Histological Typing of
Odontogenic Tumours
2nd ed. 1991. Approx. 100 pp. 142 figs. Softcover.
ISBN 3-540-54142-X

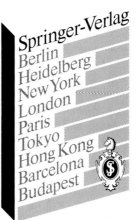

Springer-Verlag
Berlin
Heidelberg
New York
London
Paris
Tokyo
Hong Kong
Barcelona
Budapest

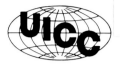

Union Against Cancer

B. Spiessl, O. H. Beahrs, P. Hermanek,
R. V. P. Hutter, O. Scheibe, L. H. Sobin,
G. Wagner (Eds.)

TNM Atlas

Illustrated Guide to the TNM/pTNM Classification of Malignant Tumours

Illustrations by U. Kerl-Jentzsch, J. Kühn

3rd ed. 1989. Corr. reprint 1990. XIX, 343 pp. 452 figs. and an insert with summaries of the T and N definitions by site. Softcover. ISBN 3-540-17721-3

The TNM classification of malignant tumours has the following objectives:
- to help the clinician determine the prognosis,
- to help the clinician in the planning of treatment,
- to assist in evaluating the results of treatment,
- to facilitate the exchange of information among treatment centres, and
- to contribute to the continuing investigation of human cancer.

The **TNM Atlas** is designed as an aid for the practical application of the TNM classification system. The corrected reprint includes the latest FIGO changes in the classification for corpus uteri and vulva carcinoma and a new insert with summaries of the T and N definitions by site.

P. Hermanek, L. H. Sobin (Eds.)

TNM Classification of Malignant Tumours

4th fully rev. ed. 1987. 2nd corr. reprint 1991. XVIII, 197 pp. Softcover. ISBN 3-540-17366-8

The TNM System is the most widely used classification of the extent of growth and the spread of cancer. Specific changes in the fourth edition include:
- elimination of all differences between the AJCC (American Joint Committee on Cancer) and the UICC TNM classifications of head and neck tumours and lung tumours,
- revision of the T classifications of esophageal and gastric carcinomas based on Japanese studies,
- modification of the classification of colorectal tumours to provide direct congruence with the Dukes' classification and allow for a finer degree of subdivision,
- redrafting in collaboration with FIGO of the FIGO classification of gynecological tumours in the format of TNM, and
- addition of TNM classification for sites not previously covered in earlier UICC editions.

D. K. Hossfeld (Chairman), C. D. Sherman, R. R. Love,
F. X. Bosch (Eds.)

Manual of Clinical Oncology

5th ed. 1990. XIV, 391 pp. 88 figs. 69 tabs. Softcover. ISBN 3-540-52769-9

The UICC **Manual of Clinical Oncology** has become a basic textbook for all students and practitioners. It gives concise, clear information on the concepts and underlying principles which govern optimal cancer prevention, diagnosis and treatment. The manual focuses intentionally on basic aspects and does not go into details of therapy, which are ever changing and controversial.
The fifth, fully revised edition has new chapters on carcinogenesis and prevention as well as many new tables and figures. The text is easy to understand and covers the basic and clinical biology of cancer in all its breadth.

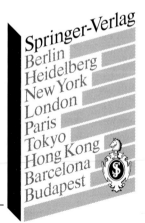

Springer-Verlag
Berlin
Heidelberg
New York
London
Paris
Tokyo
Hong Kong
Barcelona
Budapest